Acta Neurochirurgica
Supplements

Editor: H.-J. Steiger

Mechanisms of Secondary Brain Damage from Trauma and Ischemia

Recent Advances of our Understanding

Edited by
A. Baethmann, J. Eriskat, J. Lehmberg, and N. Plesnila

Acta Neurochirurgica
Supplement 89

SpringerWienNewYork

Prof. Dr. A. Baethmann
Institut für Chirurgische Forschung, Ludwig-Maximilians-Universität München, München, Germany

Dr. J. Eriskat
Neurochirurgische Klinik, Universität Würzburg, Würzburg, Germany

Dr. J. Lehmberg
Neurochirurgische Klinik, Unviersität Freiburg, Freiburg, Germany

Dr. N. Plesnila
Institut für Chirurgische Forschung, Ludwig-Maximilians-Universität München, München, Germany

Printed in Austria
Springer-Verlag Wien New York is a part of Springer Science+Business Media,
springeronline.com

Typesetting: Asco Typesetters, Hong Kong
Printing: A. Holzhausen, A-1140 Wien
Binding: Fa. Papyrus, A-1100 Wien

Printed on acid-free and chlorine-free bleached paper

SPIN: 10985786

Library of Congress Cataloging-in-Publication Data

International Symposium on Mechanisms of Secondary Brain Damage (7th : 2001 : Mauls, Italy)
Mechanisms of secondary brain damage from trauma and ischemia : recent advances of our understanding : proceedings of 7th International Symposium on Mechanisms of Secondary Brain Damage, Mauls, Italy / edited by A. Baethmann . . . [et al.].
p. ; cm. – (Acta neurochirurgica. Supplements, ISSN 0065-1419 ; 89)
Includes bibliographical references and index.
ISBN 3-211-20932-8 (alk. paper)
1. Brain damage – Congresses. 2. Cerebral ischemia – Complications – Congresses. 3. Spinal cord – Wounds and injuries – Complications – Congresses. 4. Head – Wounds and injuries – Complications – Congresses. I. Title: Proceedings of 7th International Symposium on Mechanisms of Secondary Brain Damage, Mauls, Italy. II. Baethmann, A. III. Title. IV. Acta neurochirurgica. Supplement ; 89.
[DNLM: 1. Brain Damage, Chronic – etiology – Congresses. 2. Brain Ischemia – complications – Congresses. 3. Craniocerebral Trauma – complications – Congresses. WL 354 I616m 2004]
RC387.5.I49 2003
617.4′81044—dc22
2004048154

With partly coloured Figures

ISSN 0065-1419
ISBN 3-211-20932-8 Springer Verlag Wien New York

Preface

The international interdisciplinary gathering of top level clinical and laboratory scientists in Mauls, Italy has developed from its beginning in 1984 into a fruitful tradition where worldwide experts active and knowledgeable in *cerebral ischemia and trauma* convene for update and exchanges of their most recent clinical and experimental findings and concepts. These meetings have, of course, experienced shifts in emphasis from the past until now, corresponding to the most actual developments, which were fascinating clinicians and laboratory scientists alike. The current *Supplement* of *Acta Neurochirurgica* is an example in case. Its virtue as before is that authors contribute articles in a review-like manner on their own field of research, according to the platform presentations at the meeting as indispensable basis for a spirited discussion of the expert attendants.

The present proceedings again have subheads with a spectrum from the basic sciences to patient practice. For a change *secondary brain damage* is introduced this time by a philosophical analysis on *relevance of knowledge* by a well-known philosopher of the University of Munich. The subsequent chapters contribute to the actual understanding of molecular- and cell-biological phenomena underlying or activated in *secondary brain damage*, emphasizing the availability of novel procedures as *gene profiling*, the discovery of new molecules as BID or pathways, respectively of *neuronal cells on the road to suicide* triggered by trauma or ischemia. Conversely, also the *survival of neuronal cells* injured by trauma or ischemia is discussed with regard to the support provided by neurotrophins.

The breathtaking developments of the molecular-genetic and -biological armamentarium notwithstanding, scientists driven to solve remaining problems of *secondary brain damage* by using animals with genetic deletions must be aware of the shortcomings of these novel technologies. Further, while it is no question that *ischemia* constitutes the most important factor of *secondary brain damage* in brain trauma, as acknowledged from the beginning of these workshops in Mauls, the significance of *inflammation* is all but clear. Although *inflammatory* phenomena are seen in trauma and ischemia of the brain, as activation of white blood cells with emigration into the tissue presumably enhancing damage, *inflammatory cells* may have beneficial properties as well. The chapter on the *Janus-face of inflammation* is analyzing this ambiguity.

The exploration of novel cell-biological mechanisms on a molecular or more systemic basis causing *apoptotic* cell death, *inflammation*, or *regeneration*, provide useful objectives for therapeutical interventions expected to be more specific than the present treatment modalities. This point is particularly important with regard to the deplorable situation that no drug is so far available in the hospital notwithstanding the enormous clinical and laboratory efforts. The Proceedings report new results with therapeutical promise, e.g. to interfere with the powerful proteolytic enzymes of neuronal cells (*caspases*), which definitely are proven now to have a causal function in neuronal cell death. Moreover, discussions of *secondary brain damage* are never comprehensive without up-to-date information on the mechanisms of how injured brain tissue responds to a lesion, specifically how scar formation influences regeneration.

As before, the actual state of controlled clinical drug trials assumes a major role. Specific reports are focusing on the seemingly unsolvable problem of drug trials in traumatic brain injury, specifically why the enormous efforts were all failing to identify the benefit of an agent, which under laboratory conditions is effective. Hence, clinicians are concerned of how to overcome the prevailing barrier to obtain satisfactory results or, at least, reliable explanations of the continuing dilemma. The pervasiveness of this fundamental problem makes experts increasingly wondering, whether radically different approaches are required. One attempt could be to study by far greater numbers of cases than recruited until now. This, however, would require to sacrifice valuable information on individual patients or, to identify surrogate endpoints. The Proceedings provide an impressive analysis of this conundrum which, however, is not restricted to the underlying causes but also delivers encouragement and suggestions for future improvements.

One factor which could be responsible for the problem is the lack of standardization of the management and care, which in fact comprises all the currently available treatment. Efforts were considered worthwhile, therefore, to carry out a *prospective system analysis of the patient management and care* in severe head injury with beginning of data collection at the prehospital scene immediately after the accident. Thereby, valuable information was gathered on how efficient the routine management is to prevent *secondary brain damage*. The results on standardization of treatment during this critical phase may be useful also for the planning of clinical drug trials. The findings of this population-based study, supported by the German Federal Government are impressive, as far as the technical standards and management qualities are concerned as shown, e.g. by the *prehospital rescue*, *promptness of hospital admission*, and *subsequent diagnosis and treatment*. This optimistic interpretation is based on findings that, e.g. the combination of head injury with peripheral trauma (*polytrauma*) does not worsen outcome in comparison with isolated head injury of the same severity – provided the polytrauma patient does not have risk factors, as a poor blood pressure. Another indicator of the management qualities is that the time span until conclusion of acute care (defined as admission to the *operation theater* or *intensive care unit*, respectively) per se does not affect outcome. Accordingly, patients with duration of acute care of 3 hrs were not better off than the those with 6 hrs from secondary hospital admission when neurosurgical care was not available in the primary trauma hospital. Both, the lack of additional risk from polytrauma *per se* as well as the high level of care during the acute phase serving as quality indicators may demonstrate substantial progress of the treatment including organization and management.

In conclusion, the proceedings may help again newcomers of *secondary brain damage*, interested in neurotrauma and cerebral ischemia to become familiar with the most exciting advances in the field in a comprehensive manner. The well balanced contributions of the laboratory and clinic illustrate again the enormous significance of the dialogue between both fields, ultimately for the benefit of patients. It is our hope that this publication contributes further to a better understanding of *secondary brain damage* from trauma and ischemia as basis to develop more effective treatment including drugs. Finally, outcome from trauma and ischemia of the brain and spinal cord in the future should not be determined anymore by the manifestations of *secondary damage* but only by the nature and severity of the primary insult.

It is a great pleasure to acknowledge support by the sponsors of the VIIth International Mauls Symposium and publication of its Proceedings by the Bayer AG Wuppertal, Laboratoires Fournier, Daix France, the Research Consortium *Neurotraumatologie und Neuropsychologische Rehabilitation* at the University of Munich sponsored by the Federal Ministry for Education of Research in Germany and, finally, the *Verein zur Durchführung Wissenschaftlicher Tagungen* of the Institute for Surgical Research, University of Munich. The continuing support of Springer Vienna-New York and, last but not least, the secretarial assistance by Helga Kleylein and Heidi Mehne are gratefully acknowledged.

A. Baethmann
J. Eriskat
J. Lehmberg
N. Plesnila

Contents

Listed in Current Contents

Secondary brain damage – the basic sciences

Acta Neurochir (2004) [Suppl] 89: 3–7

Knowledge matters

W. Vossenkuhl

Institute of Philosophy, Ludwig-Maximilians-University of Munich, Munich, Germany

Usefulness and knowledge

Common sense tells us that it is unreasonable to strive for things which are costly without paying and which are of no use at all. It would not be useful, e.g., to research the exact weight of King Henry VIII. Nor would it make sense to investigate whether the one-pronged fork was really invented by Herr Schnabel[1] and not by anybody else. Using research-funds for such purposes would be most unreasonable as everybody might agree.

But Common sense is far from always being reasonable itself. The maxim 'useless' equals 'unreasonable' very often goes wrong. It is indeed wrong whenever its contraposition – 'reasonable' equals 'useful' – is wrong too. Under moral conditions it is wrong most of the time to identify the reasonable and the useful. Our conscience tells us that the useful, even if it is for free, won't always go with the moral. One the other hand there are lots of things which are of no use whatever but nevertheless do appeal to us and seem to be reasonable to be achieved like, e.g., finding the biggest prime-number, writing poems or playing the piano. By the way, if the maxim 'useless' equals 'unreasonable' was true in general all the research done in the Humanities would be unreasonable too because it has no measurable or quantifiable use.

For a long time the Sciences and of course engineering were not bothered by the maxim 'useless' equals 'unreasonable'. Their use, in particular the use of their research was evident. They could easily claim to produce useful and therefore reasonable knowledge. This was obvious from the development of industrial powers and civilizational prosperity.

I'm using the past-tense here as the Sciences recently were not only criticized but again by Common sense argument – made responsible for the terrible ecological shape of the world. It seems as if scientific knowledge is useful and prone to turn out unreasonable or even dangerous at the same time. Indeed, nothing could be more unreasonable or even mad but to endanger the natural conditions of life on earth.

This brief sketch shows that from a Common sense perspective both the Sciences and the Humanities may produce unreasonable knowledge, where the further is potentially dangerous and the latter more or less innocuous. These are judgements of value publicly present and most influential in Western societies in a variety of different ideologically biased groups. None of these groups, by the way, believes that both the Sciences and the Humanities are useless. This is most deplorable because the irrationality of these judgements of value would become plainly evident if their partisans applied them to the Sciences and the Humanities simultaneously.

Judgements of value presuppose purposes and utilities. Utilities enable us to ascribe values to something. This does make sense in economics. But if the utilities are inadequate and suit their subject matter like the adjective 'gracile' does a heavy-weight champion the judgements of value are wrong. All ideologies are built on wrong judgements of value.

Inadequate utilities of boundless scientific progress like, e.g., the deliverance from all evils of mankind, as it were, ideas born from 19th Century enthusiastic scientism, led to ideological attitudes towards the Sciences.

[1] A person invented by Erich Kästner, the poet, in his Lyrische Hausapotheke.

Scientism, i.e. the belief in the liberating powers of scientific knowledge, is mistaken and like all enthusiasm causes its own frustration.

The delusions of scientism which are modern versions of post-enlightenment frenzy enthusiasm should be taken to be social mischief. We best avoid it if we estimate the usefulness of the Sciences with great care and caution. Best of all would be not to estimate both the Sciences and the Humanities primarily according to their respective usefulness but with respect to their cognitive values and achievements. If we really want to avoid prejudices or ideological attitudes we better observe this maxim.

But of course public funds are still granted according to the usefulness of expected knowledge. Shouldn't we find it curious if not alarming that research grants and technophobia are based on the very same beliefs with only reversed signs.

Technology assessment

It would be naive to suppose that it is enough to avoid prejudice and to criticise scientism in order to render to the public an adequate view of the Sciences and their achievements. Public irritations and worries caused by disappointed scientism are just too big presently. Ecological disasters fill in a long list which implicitly seems to be an accusation of science and technology: from Seveso the Bhopal, from Harrisburg to Tsernobyl. Ecological disasters or almost-disasters keep being as eagerly watched by the public as major political events. Science has become political this way.

The weekly news about disasters encroach upon people's minds causing anxieties and insecurity. Who will not be impressed and open for viable alternatives? Erwin Chargaff, the former biologist who criticizes the Sciences, proposed their abolition to avoid their great risks. Is this a sound proposal? In the vein of its logic the gazelles had to abolish the lions and the economists had to abandon the market to cope with their respective risks. Nature and human society are full of risks. They got to be controlled as their causes cannot be done away with.

No doubt, the risks of new technologies must be assessed. But it would be wholly besides the point to assign all responsibility for ecological disasters to the Sciences. Their causes are complex and manifold comprising individual failure and lack of control in the face of an immense number, diversity and densed allocation of technologies. Technology assessment may help avoid negligence born from ignorance towards risks and dangers.

I am all for technology assessment but I suspect that the political hopes going with it are too big. To calculate the risks of technologies is based on a rather limited amount of knowledge similar to what banks know about their customers borrowing money. The banks' risks are normally balanced by the customers' credit worthiness and securities. Their losses of money are compensated by equivalent values which are available beforehand. But there is no equivalent compensation for technological risks. Monetary value does not cover qualitative damages of health and environment. All calculations of risks nevertheless are bound to assume monetary equivalents for all types of damages. But their quantities should not be confused with the damages as they really occur. Most importantly, the calculation of risks should never be mistaken with mastering the probabilities of possible damage. Knowledge of risks never constrains the probability of disaster.

Take, e.g., a game of dice. Casting a five is as probable as casting a six, that is to say 1/6. But casting either a five or a six double the probability to 1/3. Now imagine two risks in a game of losing with either a five or a six where losing with a five is a serious drawback compared to losing with a six. In this game the greater risk is as probable as the lesser. And the probability of both risks taken as a mutually exclusive alternative again doubles the probabilities of each. This game shows that calculating risks won't tame the probability of the greater loss.

We should not be mislead by the real achievements of technology assessment. It will never control the probabilities of possible disasters. The security which cannot be offered by technology will not be made available by technology assessment either. Knowledge of possible consequences and side effects of technologies must be integrated into the scientific claims and standards of technological research and development. Security will be brought about primarily by those who design, develop and produce technologies.

Belief in technology assessment may have a soothing effect similar to the provisions taken by that person who did not want to run the risk of being kidnapped on a flight. He called Lufthansa asking for information about the probability of a passanger being on board carrying a bomb. Very low probability indeed, he was told. He then investigated the probability of two passengers being on board both carrying a bomb. Completely improbable, they said. He then decided to carry a bomb himself, just in case. Of course, he was wholly ignorant about the probability of himself or somebody else carrying a bomb being higher than the probability of either one carrying a bomb. He didn't lower his risk of being kidnapped. It remained the same as before.

Technology assessment should not be burdened by too great expectations nor should it be used politically to quiet public anxieties. Further, technology assessment should take special interest in the human and social quality of risks. This can be brought about by the moral analysis of the consequences and side-effects of technologies.

Moral analysis

The public attitude towards the Sciences has changed. Euphemistically it has been described as being conditioned by a 'problem of acceptance'. But the mutual relation between the Sciences and the Humanities has changed as well. The former and the latter are both present in the discourse about moral issues in the Sciences, in the Humanities and in public life. The Humanities are asked, by politicians specially, to offer orientational guidelines to enable the Sciences to determine the limits of their research and the admissible risks of their methods and aims. The need for moral analysis is undoubted.

But it is not clear how moral analysis should be able to offer orientation to the Sciences. First, the need for orientation is not unique in the Sciences. It is a general phenomenon of life. There is always a need for orientation whenever we try to balance our aspirations and powers with our moral obligations. The need for orientation means that we want to know if our aims and actions are good and responsible. Ethics is the type of analysis that tries to find an appropriate balance between individual interests, obligations and public responsibilities.

Ethics is conservative in judging what we should do now and tomorrow by following principles which were valid long before. The validity of these judgements presupposes reliable principles. Whatever changes at will is not reliable. Ethics would be unable to offer reliable judgements without being conservative.

But ethics was always in trouble with its conservatism because the old principles were rarely sufficient to solve the new problems. The respect for life and property, the principle of equality, the principles of justice and fairness, and individual freedom are indeed principles we would not like to be changed or compromised. We nevertheless are in need of new principles for the protection of nature, principles which help us follow those older principles we hold deer under the present and changed conditions of life. We understand, e.g., that respect for human life is finally not to be realized if the life of other creatures is not respected too. This comes down to something like an ethical revolution. The last revolutionary change similar to this one was the proposition of the principle of equality in 18th Century Enlightenment.

Ethics is not a closed kanon of principles. It is loyal to its older principles but is always in need of orientation too. It looks out for new or supplementary rules and criteria to bring our aspirations, conduct and obligations back into moral balance again. Of course, there is no agreement in ethics on the right principles and criteria of conduct. Rather, there is vast disagreement as the discussions on abortion and euthanasia show. There is no consensus on the value of life, nor on the licence to kill.

But ethics follows a general theoretical obligation to look for criteria to cope with disagreement on principles within its own domain in a rational way. Our own individual disagreements on values should not determine ethical analysis. Otherwise ethics could never claim to offer reliable judgements. Ethics must not settle with value-conflicts if it subscribes to the obligations of rational argument.

On the other hand, ethics cannot and should not make anybody accept or disapprove of certain values authoritatively. Rather, ethics asks each person to determine her own beliefs and aims. Because we can only be responsible for what we are up to on our own. Responsibility presupposes autonomy and self-determination. Therefore self-orientation is our duty if we claim to be morally competent beings at all. To expect unique and generally binding orientation from moral analysis confuses ethics with ideology.

But if each scientist is asked to determine his own conduct anyway why does individual morality not suffice in doing science? Why do we need an ethics of science? Because the risks of doing research are just too big for the individual scientist's personal responsibility.

Now, how is ethical orientation in the Sciences possible? Through critical ethical analysis of the values, aspirations and consequences of research. The debate in environmental and medical ethics are paradigmatic here. New types of analysis, like, e.g., Public Choice

Theory and the Theory of Collective Action are being developed to solve the problems of a fair allocation and use of public goods. Finally, ethical analysis has to take place within the Sciences if scientists want to realize self-orientation. Ethics only offers proposals and models of analysis but no ready-made solutions.

But if moral problems of science and technology should be solved it will only be possible co-operatively. Ethical analysis is asked to take kindly to the particular ethical problems in the Sciences. Any abstract recommendations won't do. Ethical expertise will only be available for scientists after a process of mutual learning and information between those who do ethics and those who do science. Again, medical ethics and its achievements of mutual learning offer an example to be recommended.

Dialogue and readability

But mutual learning and an exchange of information is bound to overcome serious obstacles. Scientists and other academic professionals, indeed all those who do research work, are speaking in different tongues. Its a Babylonian confusion going on with very little knowledge of the key concepts, the basic methods, the overall framework and scientific perspectives valid in other fields. Knowledge in one field often seems wholly bizarre and virtually nonsensical from a detached view-point. It may sound like Karl Valentin's "scientific chat": "Rain is a prismatoidical disaggregation of airlike miasmatic catalectic vibriones ..."

If something doesn't make sense to me how could I take it to be reasonable? We normally hold something to be unreasonable if we cannot tell the difference, whether it really is or only seems to be reasonable. On the other hand, we hesitate to make the reasonableness of all knowledge depend on our subjective competence of understanding. Because other people's knowledge is not supervenient on our own. Nevertheless we are bound to claim that reasonable knowledge must be *transparent*, i.e., it should in principal be open and accessible to rational judgement. In order to be transparent any representation of knowledge has to be *readable*.

For reasonable knowledge we cannot do away with the claim of transparence. But some might see the danger lurking that transparence gives rise to making the mediocre the measure of the reasonable. I wouldn't be bothered because the chance for mediocrity is small if all of those who have to offer cognitive achievements communicate their results in a readable way, readable i.e., at least on basis of some general academic training. If scientific accomplishments become readable again – as they used to be until about three or four decades ago – the Sciences' contributions for a better understanding of the world will become obvious even for those who are presently full of doubts. In the last analysis the reasonableness of all knowledge is indicated by its substantive share in an improved and more comprehensive understanding of world and nature.

We need Übersicht, i.e. good observation of what is going on in science and technology to avoid prejudice and mutual ignorance. We should be able to learn from each other and thus do our duty to obviate any further growth of techno- and scientophobia. Of course, we must first communicate in order to straighten out or own relations. There is still a lot of prejudice within the scientific community, a vicious circle as it seems and a road block if we should ever come to learn from each other. And mutual prejudice within the scientific community is growing the more the domains of knowledge are drifting apart from each other. Besides the problem of transparence mutual learning has to overcome the problems born from the speeding growth of knowledge in all fields.

This makes it more and more difficult to decide about the minimal content of mutual knowledge. To strive for encyclopedic knowledge is definitely a lost option. But the minimal content of knowledge which is truly relevant is not easy to describe. There are at least two criteria of minimal content: first, it must be sufficient for ethical analysis, i.e., we need an understanding of possible risks and consequences of knowledge; second, it must be good enough to improve our picture of world and nature.

But again, mutual learning and communication will only be possible if the Sciences offer readable knowledge, if the representations of cognitive content and scientific achievements are minimally transparent. A handy and unassuming test for minimal transparence is to understand answers to simple questions like "what are you doing?" We might in the end be able to catch a glimpse of the universe of knowledge which used to be the reference of the name 'university'.

By the way, readability and transparence do not come down to popularization. Something difficult is not to be explained if you just avoid the difficult bits. Journalists are supposed to popularize knowledge by making it simple and easy to understand. Transparence and readability preserve the basic structures, the key notions and the reach of knowledge. Otherwise it will neither enable ethical analysis nor give an improved picture of the world.

Readability and transparence of scientific knowledge are not only wanted by the members of the scientific community. There are members of parliament and bureaucrats in political institutions to decide about the funding of the Sciences and academic institutions. They have an interest in the transparence of scientific knowledge too. If the cognitive content of research is not to be communicated how will public funding ever be guided by rational insight?

The Sciences, the Humanities and the Arts offer the only human ways of understanding the world. The reasonableness of knowledge, as I claimed above, depends on its contribution to an improved and more comprehensive picture of the world as a whole. But if the increase and particularization of knowledge impairs its communication, scientific knowledge will not contribute to an understanding of the world. The less it contributes the more its enhancement is unreasonable.

Please note, its not its quantity which makes knowledge unreasonable but our inability to discriminate between reasonable and unreasonable knowledge. In other words, we are unable to give a perspicuous and structured account of knowledge, structured, as it were, to fit an intelligible picture of the world. But what shall we do with unreasonable knowledge? We all know what we do, the only thing to be done with it: it is put in alphabetic order, catalogued and administrated in libraries where the empty spaces are dwindling away. Thus knowledge becomes antiquarian before its cognitive value has become apparent, before we had the chance to become more knowledgeable.

I started off pleading not to confuse the reasonable with the useful and judge scientific knowledge primarily according to its cognitive value. From contemporary techno- and scientophobia we learn that the Sciences are vulnerable to ideological prejudice if its use determines its value. Finally I mentioned some of the difficulties to judge the cognitive value of scientific knowledge and tried to clarify some of the criteria of reasonable knowledge. In between I dealt with the need for orientation and ethical analysis.

I do believe that these areas of problems are intimately connected. Just observe the chain of conditionals from its end: if we don't perceive the value of scientific knowledge for our understanding of the world, we cannot tell the difference between reasonable and unreasonable knowledge; if we cannot discern this difference we are unable to develop a reasonable picture of the world as a whole; if we don't have such a picture available we are in need of orientation in whatever we research and investigate. In this case we lack Übersicht, we have no survey. The need for ethical analysis seen from this angle is nothing but a lack of reasonable knowledge.

But of course, reasonable knowledge is not easily available. It might nevertheless be easier to get than knowledge of the notorious "Schleswig-Holstein affair". In the House of Commons Lord Palmerston, then prime minister, was asked about the "Schleswig-Holstein affair". Palmerston explained that there were only three people who ever knew what the "Schleswig-Holstein affair" was all about: Bismarck, himself of course, and a German philosopher. Bismarck was dead, he had forgotten and the German philosopher went mad thinking about it.

Correspondence: W. Vossenkuhl, Institute of Philosophy, Ludwig-Maximilians-University of Munich, D-80539 Munich, Germany. e-mail: Vossenkuhl@lrz.uni-muenchen.de

Acta Neurochir (2004) [Suppl] 89: 9–13

Printed in Austria

Gene profiling – chances and challenges

G. Enders

Institute for Surgical Research, Klinikum Grosshadern, Munich, Germany

Summary

Microarray analysis has been emerged as a tool to characterize the overall reaction of cells in culture or tissue to different stimuli e.g. stressful events by analysing bulk RNA present at a particular time point. It has supplemented or even replaced more traditional methods like cDNA-bank sequencing or conventional differential display. The commercial availability of several different precoated arrays and the ease of handling has supported the broad distribution of this new technique.

The basic protocol involves the hybridization of complementary strands of labelled DNA or RNA from cells/tissue with representations of known genes spotted onto a solid support (nylon, glass). Labelling can be radioactive ($P^{32/33}$), by a hapten group (biotin, digoxigenin, aminoallyl) or by fluorescent (Cy3, Cy5 etc.) nucleotides. Detection is performed by autoradiography, chemiluminescence or fluorescence scanning. There are different setups of arrays available: either known genes/gene-groups (apoptosis, cytokines etc.) are spotted as PCR fragments, plasmids or synthetic oligonucleotides or representations of the known genome are directly synthesized as short sequence tags of 20–70 oligonucleotides on glass chips. The latter allow the identification of newly expressed genes whereas the former deal with known genes. Ideally, the intensity of the signal can be correlated with the relative expression of a known gene and allows the comparison with a standard. Problems arise from the quality of the sample material, the standardization of the protocols and the data management. Nevertheless, gene profiling by cDNA-arrays will definitely be integrated into routine screening programs.

Keywords: Gene expression; DNA-Array.

It is the basic understanding of biology, that thousands of genes and their products in a given organism function in a complicated way to adapt the system to external and internal stimuli. In an experimental systems this reaction of an organ or cell system can be followed by measuring the amount and quality of mRNA synthesized in response to a known trigger. This has conventionally been analysed by Northern blotting, RNAse protection or dot blot analysis. More recently the possibility and ease of handling of the polymerase chain reaction has introduced RT-PCR into the experimental and diagnostic repertoire. Although all this methods are accurate and stringent they all bear the inherent problem that one surveys only a restricted amount of genes and has to know exactly which gene one is looking for. This makes it reasonable to oversee important candidate genes involved in regulation. To circumvent this, micro array analysis has emerged as a powerful, high throughput tool to measure the relative expression of thousands of individual genes in parallel under different experimental conditions [6, 13] or between different pathological entities.

The experimental basis is to compare mRNA expressed in one subset of cells/tissue with a control set. So the experimental steps include isolation of the RNA of interest in form of total or mRNA, labelling of it and hybridizing it to an array of pieces of DNA with known sequence. *The basic technology* includes hybridization of labelled cDNA from a target sample with an array of complementary DNA or oligonucleotides of known sequence spotted onto a solid support matrices like nylon, plastic or glass. For this total RNA or mRNA must be isolated from the target cells or the tissue sample of interest. This is usually an easy approach when dealing with isolated cells in culture but not trivial with organ samples. Since cells in culture can be exposed to a particular stimulus all at once the reaction can be assumed to be uniform and differences in RNA expression reflect the specific answer to the stimulus. In complex tissue samples on the other hand it is always difficult to answer specific questions since different cell types/areas of an organ may react

---

The author apologizes that due to the enormous increase in publications using microarray analysis only a small sample of relevant citations could be included.

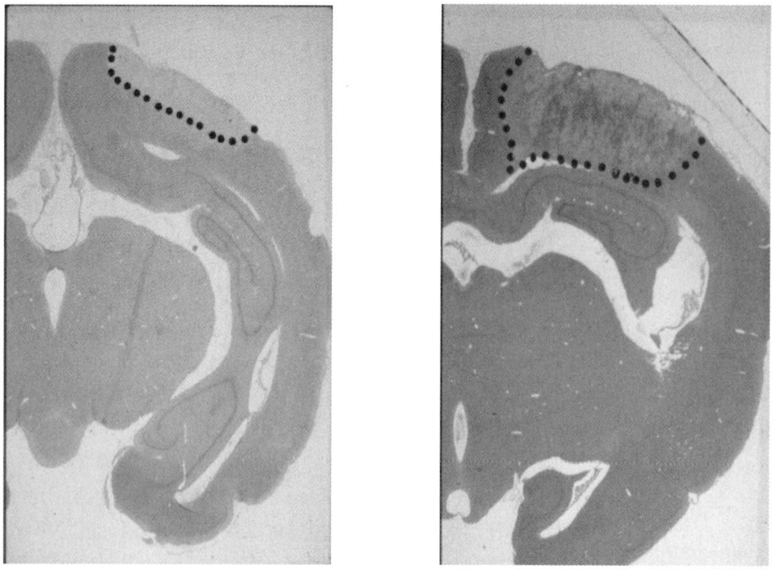

Fig. 1. Histologic section of a brain after cold injury. The dotted line gives the extend of necrosis immediately (a) and 24 hours (b) after the injury. The zone adjacent to the initial necrosis is the area of interest for the analysis of expressed genes by e.g. gene-array. (Histology kindly provided by Prof. A. Baethmann/Dr. J. Eriskat)

differently. To give an example, the gene profiling of new and specific genes expressed after an initial insult in the brain could be laborious and even show no difference, when the samples contain cells with different sensitivity to the injury. So only the isolation of the specific areas/cells allows to ask precise questions. This can be illustrated by an example of an injury to the brain, where after the primary damage a secondary brain damage may develop in the area around the primary necrotic tissue (penumbra, Fig. 1). This area is of special interest since the follow up of genes expressed could give valuable insights into the developmental regulation of the tissue damage and may offer therapeutic clues. Other examples where the discrimination of gene expression is important are differentiation between cancerous and normal or inflamed and control tissue. In all these cases one needs a very accurate separation between the samples of interest and proper controls. For this accurate decision sophisticated devices (laser capture) exist which allow the isolation of the samples of interest from the rest on slightly counterstained histologic preparations [7]. It is quite obvious that the amount of RNA which can be isolated from such small samples is limited and sometimes further analysis needs amplification steps. There are amplification procedures for RNA as well as cDNA around but due to the problem of non linear amplification of the template the results might be hard to interpret. Direct labelling of the cDNA using reverse transciptase and properly labelled nucleotides is the method of choice when enough RNA is available. Protocols vary from 100 ng to 2 μg RNA as the amount of starting material required. Labelled nucleotides include radioactive, fluorescent, biotin, digoxigenin or aminoallyl-tagged dNTP. The choice of label depends on preferences and the equipment of the laboratory for detection after hybridization. There might be differences in the processivity of the reverse transciptase depending on the alteration in the different nucleotides. After labelling, this template is now ready for hybridization to an array of DNA or oligonucleotides spotted onto a solid support.

Arrays commercially available differ in at least three points: the genetic information used on the array, the technology of application and the material for the array support. The genes can be represented on the array as plasmid DNA, PCR-products or oligonucleotides spotted or directly synthesized on the support. All of these methods have advantages and disadvantage: Plasmid DNA has the inherent problem of high background hybridization with e.g. bacterial DNA, PCR products must be highly purified but due to their length are quite specific and oligonucleotides must have a certain length and need a lot of bioinformatics for their design. With this regard nucleotides from 50 to 70 base length have been shown to be reasonably specific and might be the method of choice because they can easily and well defined be synthesized and spotted. In addition defined regions and multiple segments of a particular gene can be applied which serves as a good control for mispriming. The more advanced technology of the synthesis of overlapping nucleotides representing the total known genome directly on the glass support as developed and sold by Affymetrix gives an excellent overview but is very expensive. In addition the test needs expensive lab equipment which is normally not in the basic setup of a routine lab.

Material for the support: Originally the arrays consisted of plasmid DNA spotted onto a regular nylon membrane. But soon after that glass arrays became available. Nylon arrays have the advantage that the basic technology for hybridization is present in routine molecular biological labs from traditional techniques like Southern, Northern or dot-blotting. In addition the tools for the detection of the hybridized signal whether you screen with a radioactive or a tagged probe and enzymatic detection including chemiluminescent substrates are available in a standard molecular biology lab. Another approach was spotting the genetic information in form of plasmid DNA, PCR-products or synthetic oligonucleotides on glass slides or even synthesizing stretches of genes as oligonucleotides directly on an activated glass support. Glass slides have the advantage that the information can be very densely spotted and that the hybridization can be done with fluorescently labelled cDNA. By using different fluorescence tags it is possible to screen a particular expression profile to be evaluated on the same array provided that a scanner/detector with the correct wavelength is available. A popular combination involves the labelling of the control sample with e.g. Cy3-dUTP and that of the experimental/stimulated samples with Cy5-dUTP. Both targets can then be mixed and hybridized on the same array. Testing it on the same array allows to bypass problems with the variability in the actual hybridization process or in the quality of the array itself.

One problem comes with the quality and reproducibility of the genetic information on the array. Thus arrays are sometimes a kind of a black box and the user relies on the information offered by the manufacturing company. That this is not a trivial problems can be seen from a recent estimate that up to 30% of arrays have been tested erroneous [4]. So proper *controls* are needed. The presence of several housekeeping genes as positive controls as well as bacterial or yeast genes as negative controls are important steps in the development of reliable standards. In addition the representation of several stretches of the same gene and the inclusion of hybridization controls by adding mismatch controls adds further certainty in the specificity and information got by this technology. The inclusion of a control by spiking the sample with a e.g. phage RNA and having the corresponding sequences on the array allows normalization and quantification of this particular sequence as well as detecting differences in the overall hybridization between different sets of arrays.

Quantification is of particular interest. Detection limit and threshold for differences are important decisions followed by an evaluation software since handling of teens of thousands of gene sequences is usually beyond the scope of manual elaboration. A difference in the hybridization signal of more than twofold is expected to represent a distinct difference in expression of this gene. As shown diagrammatically on Fig. 2 the intensity of the hybridization signal for each particular gene can be arranged in a coordinate grid. Every deviation from the diagonal axis indicates a difference between the control (x-axis) and experimental group (y-axis). A difference of more than twofold is expected

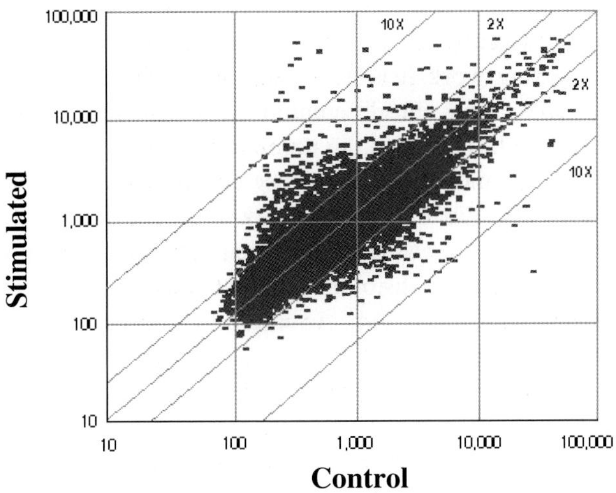

Fig. 2. Histogram of an array analysis. Relative intensities for given genes in control as well as stimulated cells are plotted. Dots on the diagonal are equally represented in controls and stimulated cells. The range for ×2 and ×10 is given as an example. Dots beyond this limit show over/under-representation of a given gene

to be of relevance. One can easily see, that even this stringent determination gives numerous differentially expressed genes. Having ~65 000 tags on the Affymetrix chip does't allow the manual evaluation. For this evaluation sophisticated computer programs have been developed including statistical programs and artificial neural networks [3, 11]. At the end total analysis needs pattern recognition as well as data mining experience is important.

So, how to make a decision on a certain experiment which array is useful for getting maximal/optimal and also meaningful results? It mostly depends on whether the goal of the experiment is to get an overview on as many as possible *known* genes or the detection of *new* genes. The former can best be answered by using an array where DNA from gene-families e.g. cytokines, adhesion molecules or expected candidate genes like stress genes, cell cycle genes or genes suspected to be involved in cancer are spotted on the array. The advantage with arrays like these is that only known genes with a defined function are represented on the array so that interpretation is more convenient. A disadvantage is that the use of these arrays will disregard the detection of new and unknown genes. Therefore, arrays are around with huge amounts of sequenced genes but also ESTs with even unknown function. The information on the human genome even allows to represent the total genome-sequence on a chip.

Examples for the different setups have proven their usefulness. So the total analysis of 65 000 genes on diseases as different as leukemia [1] has changed our view on disease classification with consequences even on the therapy [2, 8]. On the other hand after these pioneering work it is now clear that only a handful of genes allow the differentiation of leukaemia and therefore has reduced the number of genes to be analysed in clinical practice. Other examples from brain research shows that DNA-array analysis has broadened the view on tissue specific gene expression within the brain, pathopyhsiology of ischemia as well as some disease [5, 9, 10, 12, 14]. An interesting outcome from these experiments is that quite often only a handful of genes are differentially expressed making it easier for follow up studies.

Microarray technology (including oligonucleotide arrays and cDNA arrays) offers great promise to functional genomics research, and potentially transforms the diagnosis and treatment of diseases. Limitations include the paucity of RNA from small samples, the quality of RNA from medical samples, the detection limit (2X) but also the price for arrays. However, a standard protocol for microarray data analysis has yet to be established. There are attempts to standardize the procedure to make results comparable. There are also suggestions for the adoption of standards for DNA-array experiment annotation and data representation, as well as the introduction of standard experimental controls and data normalization which may even influence the reviewing process for publication (for information see internet pages). The critical assessment of microarray analysis guarantees that it will be a powerful method which finally will be part of the basic laboratory tools for analysis by which it will be possible to create important scientific progress.

References

1. Alizadeh AA, Eisen MB, Davis RE, Ma C *et al* (2000) Distinct types of diffuse large B-cell lymphoma identified by gene expression profiling. Nature 403: 503–511
2. Bittner M, Meltzer P, Chen Y *et al* (2000) Molecular classification of cutaneous malignant melanoma by gene expression profiling. Nature 406: 536–540
3. Khan J, Wei JS, Ringner M, Saal LH, Ladanyi M, Westermann F, Berthold F, Schwab M, Antonescu CR, Peterson C, Meltzer PS (2001) Classification and diagnostic prediction of cancers using gene expression profiling and artificial neural networks. Nat Med 7: 673–679
4. Knight J (2001) When the chips are down. Nature 410: 860–861
5. Li JY, Boado RJ, Pardridge WM (2001) Blood-brain barrier genomics. J Cereb Blood Flow Metab 21: 61–68
6. Lockhart DJ, Winzeler EA (2000) Genomics, gene expression and DNA arrays. Nature 405: 827–836
7. Luo L, Salunga RC, Guo H, Bittner A, Joy KC, Galindo JE, Xiao H, Rogers KE, Wan JS, Jackson MR, Erlander MG (1999) Gene expression profiles of laser-captured adjacent neuronal subtypes. Nat Med 5: 117–122, 827–836
8. Marx J (2000) Medicine. DNA arrays reveal cancer in its many forms. Science 289: 1670–1672
9. Mirnics K, Middleton FA, Lewis DA, Levitt P (2001) Analysis of complex brain disorders with gene expression microarrays: schizophrenia as a disease of the synapse. Trends Neurosci 24: 479–486
10. Mirnics K (2001) Microarrays in brain research: the good, the bad and the ugly. Nat Rev Neurosci 2: 444–447
11. Pan KH, Lih CJ, Cohen SN (2002) Analysis of DNA microarrays using algorithms that employ rule-based expert knowledge. Proc Natl Acad Sci USA 99: 2118–2123
12. Sklar P, Schwab SG, Williams NM *et al* (2001) Association analysis of NOTCH4 loci in schizophrenia using family and population-based controls. Nat Genet 28: 126–128
13. Young RA (2000) Biomedical discovery with DNA arrays. Cell 102: 9–15
14. Zirlinger M, Kreiman G, Anderson DJ (2001) Amygdala-enriched genes identified by microarray technology are restricted to specific amygdaloid subnuclei. Proc Natl Acad Sci USA 98: 5270–5275

Useful internet pages

http://microarrays.org/index.html
http://www.ncbi.nlm.nih.gov/geo
http://www.ebi.ac.uk/arrayexpress
http://www.gene-chips.com
http://www.bioinformatics.duke.edu/camda
http://www.mged.org

Correspondence: G. Enders, M.D., Institute for Surgical Research, Klinikum Grosshadern, Marchioninistr. 27, D-81366 Munchen, Germany. e-mail: enders@icf.med.uni-muenchen.de

Acta Neurochir (2004) [Suppl] 89: 15–19

Printed in Austria

Role of mitochondrial proteins for neuronal cell death after focal cerebral ischemia

N. Plesnila

Institute for Surgical Research, University of Munich, Munich, Germany

Summary

Cell death following focal cerebral ischemia has an acute and a delayed component. Delayed neuronal cell death occurs via activation of molecular signalling pathways resembling apoptosis in non-neuronal cells. Cell surface cell death receptors and damage to mitochondria or DNA initiate these pathways finally leading to DNA fragmentation and cell death. Central mediators of delayed neuronal cell death are two families of molecules: a group of cysteine aspartate proteases, called caspases, and molecules of the bcl-2 family, e.g. bcl-2, bax, and bid. Caspases initiate and execute cell death, while bcl-2 family members modulate death signalling and lead to release of pro-apoptotic molecules from the mitochondrial intermembranous space, e.g. cytochrome c and apoptosis inducing factor (AIF). Cytochrome c induces cell death by activation of caspase 9 and 3, while AIF leads to detrimental DNA damage by an capase-independent pathway. The current paper reviews recent findings dealing with pre- and post-mitochondrial cell death pathways activated by focal cerebral ischemia.

Keywords: Cerebral ischemia; Cell death; Bcl-2; Bid, AIF.

Programmed cell death is a feature of chronic and acute neurodegenerative diseases including Alzheimer's and Huntington's disease, amyotrophic lateral sclerosis (ALS), and stroke [20, 42]. It is mediated in part by caspases, a family of cysteine proteases that cleave and disassemble proteins essential for cell survival [26]. Caspases are activated during cerebral ischemia [13, 22, 36], and ischemic cell death is significantly attenuated by caspase inhibition [11] or caspase gene deletion [29].

The sequence of events leading to caspase activation has been well characterised in non-neuronal cells [33]. In these cells, Bid, a 22 kDa cytosolic member of the Bcl-2 family of pro-apoptotic proteins [37], provides one mechanism by which TNF/Fas family death receptor activation is linked to downstream events [21]. These death receptors activate caspase-8, which cleaves Bid to its truncated active form (tBid; 15 kDa) [16]. tBid targets the outer mitochondrial membrane and induces conformational changes in BAK and BAX [43] and by so doing, triggers the release of cytochrome c and apoptosis-inducing factor (AIF) into the cytosol [34, 38]. Cytochrome c together with APAF-1 and caspase-9 form the apoptosome complex, which results in activation of caspase-3 and other effector caspases which ultimately cause cell death [44]. Upon release from mitochondria AIF translocates to the nucleus where it induces DNA fragmentation by an caspase-independent, yet unknown mechanism. The importance of Bid in death receptor mediated programmed cell death and in amplification of upstream cell death signals is demonstrated by the fact that *bid* knockout mice are strongly resistant to death receptor induced hepatocellular apoptosis [40].

Similar molecular events leading to programmed cell death in non-neuronal cells have only recently been described after experimental stroke (focal cerebral ischemia), e.g., expression of cell surface death receptors of the TNF/Fas family [12, 17, 27], cleavage of caspase-8 [36] and caspase-3 [22], and release of cytochrome c from mitochondria [8]. That these molecular signalling pathways have also a therapeutic potential has been shown by the neuroprotective action of caspase inhibitors [4, 6] and by the fact that *caspase-3* knock-out mice have significantly smaller infarcts than their wild-type littermates [14].

Until recently very little was known about the mechanisms leading to release of mitochondrial proteins after cerebral ischemia, e.g. whether Bid is expressed in the brain and whether it has similar death-promoting properties as in non-neuronal cells. To explore this hypothesis, we used well-characterised models of ischemic cell death [oxygen-glucose deprivation (OGD) and middle cerebral artery occlusion

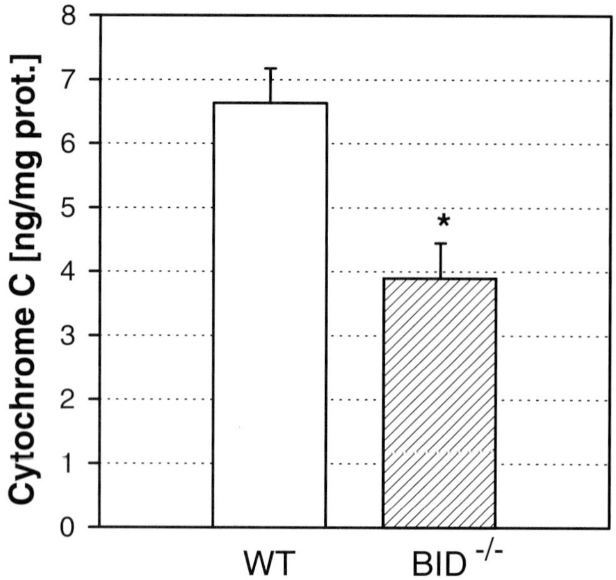

Fig. 1. Cytochrome c release after focal ischemia. Following ischemia, 41% less cytochrome c was measured by ELISA in the cytosol of Bid$^{-/-}$ mice ($n = 4$) as compared to wild type littermates ($n = 4$, $^*p < 0.03$). From [25]

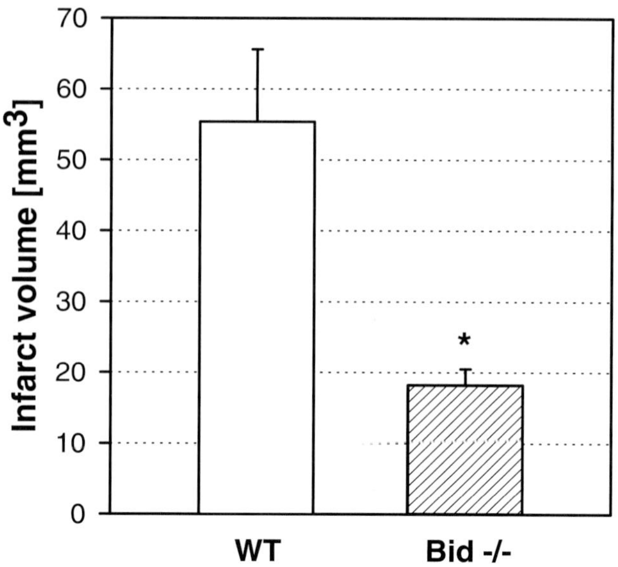

Fig. 2. Ischemic damage is reduced in Bid$^{-/-}$ mice. Infarct volume was reduced by 67% in Bid$^{-/-}$ mice as compared to wild type mice ($n = 8$ per group; $^*p < 0.01$) after 30 min middle cerebral artery occlusion and 48 hours reperfusion. From [25]

(MCAo)] to determine whether Bid is cleaved after ischemia, and whether *bid* knockout mice show neuroprotection after experimental stroke. In addition we examined the relationship between the presence of activated Bid (tBid) and cytochrome c release in adult mouse brain.

Our findings demonstrate that in the CNS, cytochrome c release in ischemic striatum from *bid*$^{-/-}$ mice is attenuated following middle cerebral artery occlusion (Fig. 1), and that caspase-3 activation is reduced after oxygen glucose deprivation in *bid*$^{-/-}$ cortical neurons [25]. As a consequence Bid deletion reduces neuronal cell death after oxygen glucose deprivation and after focal cerebral ischemia (Fig. 2) [25]. Our findings establish Bid as a critical mediator of ischemic cell death within the central nervous system. Despite strong evidence linking Bid to pore formation in the outer mitochondrial membrane and to cytosolic release of cytochrome c, cytochrome c release was not completely abrogated in cells and tissues of *bid*$^{-/-}$ mice. Release was apparently not caused by complete rupture of mitochondrial membranes as cytochrome oxidase, a mitochondrial protein, was not detected in cytosolic fractions (data not shown). Our data suggest that Bid is not the sole mechanism for cytochrome c release after cerebral ischemia. Other mechanisms and molecules may contribute to the release process, such as unique mechanisms related to Bax, Bad, Bcl-2, Bcl-X_L, oxygen radicals, MnSOD, or opening of the mitochondrial permeability transition [7, 10, 31, 32]. Furthermore, BCL-2, and BCL-w modulate cytochrome c release, and an increase in their expression could protect tissues from injury during ischemia [19, 39]. Bid and other mechanisms may also effect survival in non-neuronal cell types (e.g., astrocytes, endothelial cells, microglia) spared in ischemic *bid*$^{-/-}$ mouse brain. Further work is necessary to clarify this point. Nevertheless, the results generated using *bid*$^{-/-}$ mice convincingly demonstrate a prominent role for Bid in acute CNS injury.

Our findings concerning Bid also shed light on the signalling pathway activated in neurons after an ischemic insult. In non-neuronal cells, caspase activation can occur via a sequence of events known as type II death receptor signalling [28], in which stimulation of death receptors activates caspase-8. Caspase-8 in turn cleaves Bid to tBid. After migration to the mitochondrial membrane and interaction with Bax, tBid causes cytochrome c release from mitochondria and results in the activation of caspase-3 and other caspases. Our data show that the molecular pathway for ischemic cell death in neurons resembles the type II pathway. Caspase-8 is constitutively expressed in brain, and focal ischemia triggers its activation in vivo

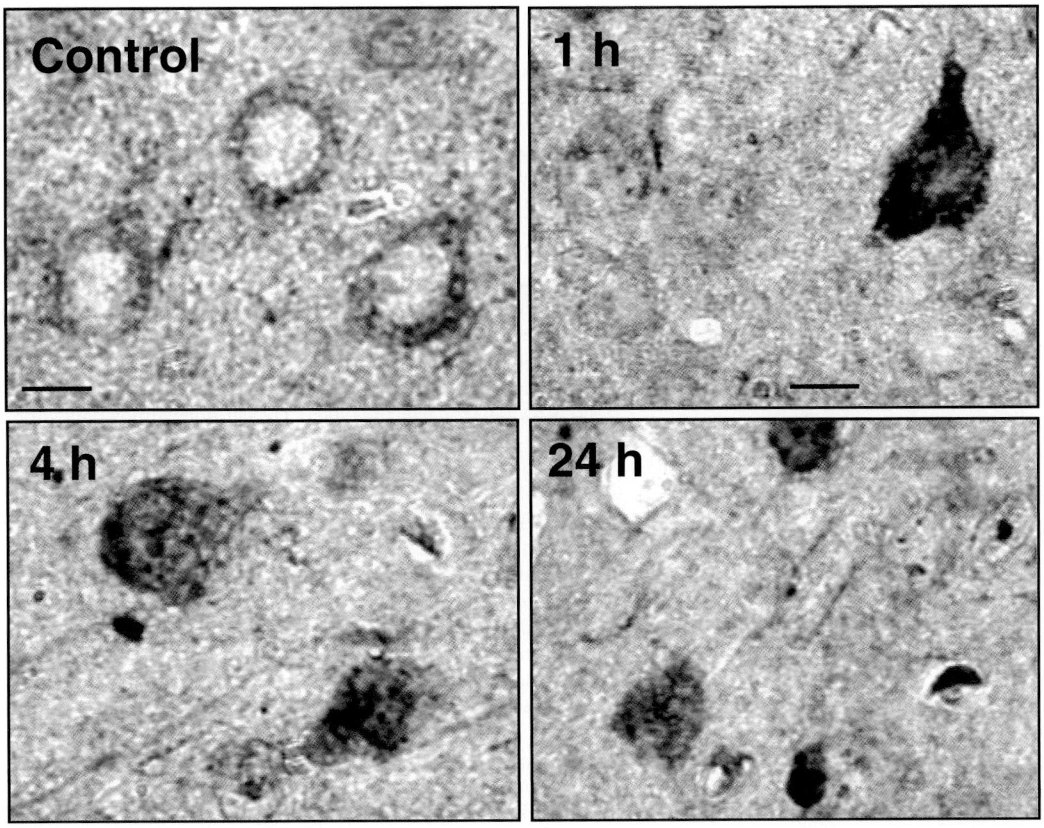

Fig. 3. AIF translocation after focal cerebral ischemia. In the cerebral cortex of sham operated mice *(Control)* AIF is only located outside the nucleus, i.e. in mitochondria. Already one hour after reperfusion from 45 min middle cerebral artery occlusion AIF translocates to the nucleus in single cells. Four and 24 hours after ischemia cells with nuclear AIF show typical signs of delayed neuronal death, e.g. nuclear condensation and fragmentation. From [24]

[36]. We have shown that caspase-8 cleaves Bid to tBid from brain homogenates (Fig. 1b). Taken together, it is likely that caspase-8, being the cysteine protease with the strongest Bid-cleaving activity, mediates Bid cleavage in the CNS [16].

Although caspase activation has been identified as a major molecular mechanism of programmed cell death, recent findings indicate the importance of additional non-caspase-dependent mechanisms [1, 2, 23]. Recently, a novel pro-apoptotic molecule, apoptosis-inducing factor (AIF), was identified [35] as a 67 kDa flavoprotein with significant homology to bacterial and plant oxidoreductases and located in the mitochondrial intermembranous space. Upon release from mitochondria, AIF migrates to the nucleus where it induces large-scale ($\sim$50 kbp) DNA fragmentation and apoptosis by a yet unknown, caspase-independent mechanism [3, 23]. Based on these assumptions AIF may be a novel factor that is released together with cytochrome c from mitochondria and leads to cell death following experimental stroke (focal cerebral ischemia). Experiments performed on primary cultured neurons after oxygen/glucose deprivation and on mouse brain tissue subjected to focal cerebral ischemia by MCAo, clearly demonstrate that apoptosis-inducing factor (AIF) was indeed released from mitochondria and translocates to the nucleus during post-ischemic neuronal cell death in vivo and in vitro (Fig. 3). AIF translocation to the nucleus was associated with apoptosis-like nuclear morphology, e.g., nuclear condensation and fragmentation, DNA damage, and with cell death, suggesting that AIF may be involved in post-ischemic neuronal cell death [24]. Counting of cytochrome c- and AIF-positive cells in ischemic brain tissue showed that the number of cell showing nuclear AIF staining outnumbered those showing mitochondrial cytochrome c release [24]. This may suggest that AIF and cytochrome c, which cause caspase-independent and caspase-dependent DNA damage downstream of mitochondria, respectively, are equally important for cell demise in cerebral ischemia. The parallel or subsequent activation of caspase-dependent/cytochrome c-mediated and caspase-independent/AIF-mediated cell death pathways may well serve as a good explanation for several previous findings after experimental stroke. For example, *caspase-3* knock-out mice show significant neuroprotection after focal ischemia [15], however, less than was anticipated based on previous studies showing impressive neuroprotection by modulation of mitochondrial proteins, e.g. by cyclosporine A [30, 41], knock-out of *bid* [25], overexpression of *sod* [9] and *bcl-2* [18].

In summary, Bid promotes cell death in the brain following focal cerebral ischemia by triggering the release of pro-apoptotic proteins from mitochondria, e.g., cytochrome c and AIF. Downstream of mitochondria not only caspases but also caspase-independent mechanisms, e.g., AIF, are responsible for DNA damage and the final execution of the cell death program. This may explain why caspase inhibitors are less neuroprotective than anticipated. Because Bid is strategically located upstream of mitochondria and triggers caspase-3 and AIF activation [5], and AIF represents a death pathway parallel to the downstream caspases 3, 6, and 7, Bid and AIF may represent attractive therapeutic targets for central nervous system diseases in which apoptotic cell death is prominent.

References

1. Cande C, Cecconi F, Dessen P, Kroemer G (2002) Apoptosis-inducing factor (AIF): key to the conserved caspase-independent pathways of cell death? J Cell Sci 115: 4727–4734
2. Cregan SP, Fortin A, MacLaurin JG, Callaghan SM, Cecconi F, Yu SW, Dawson TM, Dawson VL, Park DS, Kroemer G, Slack RS (2002) Apoptosis-inducing factor is involved in the regulation of caspase-independent neuronal cell death. J Cell Biol 158: 507–517
3. Daugas E, Susin SA, Zamzami N, Ferri KF, Irinopoulou T, Larochette N, Prevost MC, Leber B, Andrews D, Penninger J, Kroemer G (2000) Mitochondrio-nuclear translocation of AIF in apoptosis and necrosis. FASEB J 14: 729–739
4. Endres M, Namura S, Shimizu-Sasamata M, Waeber C, Zhang L, Gomez-Isla T, Hyman BT, Moskowitz MA (1998) Attenuation of delayed neuronal death after mild focal ischemia in mice by inhibition of the caspase family. J Cereb Blood Flow Metab 18: 238–247
5. Fink K, Zhu J, Namura S, Shimizu-Sasamata M, Endres M, Ma J, Dalkara T, Yuan J, Moskowitz MA (1998) Prolonged therapeutic window for ischemic brain damage caused by delayed caspase activation. J Cereb Blood Flow Metab 18: 1071–1076
6. Fink K, Zhu J, Namura S, Shimizu-Sasamata M, Endres M, Ma J, Dalkara T, Yuan J, Moskowitz MA (1998) Prolonged therapeutic window for ischemic brain damage caused by delayed caspase activation. J Cereb Blood Flow Metab 18: 1071–1076
7. Fiskum G, Murphy AN, Beal MF (1999) Mitochondria in neurodegeneration: acute ischemia and chronic neurodegenerative diseases. J Cereb Blood Flow Metab 19: 351–369
8. Fujimura M, Morita-Fujimura Y, Murakami K, Kawase M, Chan PH (1998) Cytosolic redistribution of cytochrome c after transient focal cerebral ischemia in rats. J Cereb Blood Flow Metab 18: 1239–1247
9. Fujimura M, Morita-Fujimura Y, Noshita N, Sugawara T, Kawase M, Chan PH (2000) The cytosolic antioxidant copper/zinc-superoxide dismutase prevents the early release of mitochondrial cytochrome c in ischemic brain after transient focal cerebral ischemia in mice. J Neurosci 20: 2817–2824
10. Fujimura M, Morita-Fujimura Y, Noshita N, Sugawara T, Kawase M, Chan PH (2000) The cytosolic antioxidant copper/zinc-superoxide dismutase prevents the early release of mitochondrial cytochrome c in ischemic brain after transient focal cerebral ischemia in mice. J Neurosci 20: 2817–2824
11. Hara H, Friedlander RM, Gagliardini V, Ayata C, Fink K, Huang Z, Shimizu-Sasamata M, Yuan J, Moskowitz MA (1997) Inhibition of interleukin 1beta converting enzyme family proteases reduces ischemic and excitotoxic neuronal damage. Proc Natl Acad Sci USA 94: 2007–2012
12. Harrison DC, Roberts J, Campbell CA, Crook B, Davis R, Deen K, Meakin J, Michalovich D, Price J, Stammers M, Maycox PR (2000) TR3 death receptor expression in the normal and ischaemic brain. Neuroscience 96: 147–160
13. Krajewski S, Krajewska M, Ellerby LM, Welsh K, Xie Z, Deveraux QL, Salvesen GS, Bredesen DE, Rosenthal RE, Fiskum G, Reed JC (1999) Release of caspase-9 from mitochondria during neuronal apoptosis and cerebral ischemia. Proc Natl Acad Sci USA 96: 5752–5757
14. Le DA, Wu Y, Huang Z, Matsushita K, Plesnila N, Augustinack JC, Hyman BT, Yuan J, Kuida K, Flavell RA, Moskowitz MA (2002) Caspase activation and neuroprotection in caspase-3-deficient mice after in vivo cerebral ischemia and in vitro oxygen glucose deprivation. Proc Natl Acad Sci USA 99: 15188–15193
15. Le DA, Wu Y, Huang Z, Matsushita K, Plesnila N, Augustinack JC, Hyman BT, Yuan J, Kuida K, Flavell RA, Moskowitz MA (2002) Caspase activation and neuroprotection in caspase-3-deficient mice after in vivo cerebral ischemia and in vitro oxygen glucose deprivation. Proc Natl Acad Sci USA 99: 15188–15193
16. Li H, Zhu H, Xu CJ, Yuan J (1998) Cleavage of BID by caspase 8 mediates the mitochondrial damage in the Fas pathway of apoptosis. Cell 94: 491–501
17. Martin-Villalba A, Herr I, Jeremias I, Hahne M, Brandt R, Vogel J, Schenkel J, Herdegen T, Debatin KM (1999) CD95 ligand (Fas-L/APO-1L) and tumor necrosis factor-related apoptosis-inducing ligand mediate ischemia-induced apoptosis in neurons. J Neurosci 19: 3809–3817
18. Martinou JC, Dubois-Dauphin M, Staple JK, Rodriguez I, Frankowski H, Missotten M, Albertini P, Talabot D, Catsicas S, Pietra C (1994) Overexpression of BCL-2 in transgenic mice protects neurons from naturally occurring cell death and experimental ischemia. Neuron 13: 1017–1030
19. Martinou JC, Dubois-Dauphin M, Staple JK, Rodriguez I, Frankowski H, Missotten M, Albertini P, Talabot D, Catsicas S, Pietra C (1994) Overexpression of BCL-2 in transgenic mice protects neurons from naturally occurring cell death and experimental ischemia. Neuron 13: 1017–1030
20. Mattson MP (2000) Apoptosis in neurodegenerative disorders. Nature Reviews Molecular Cell Biology 1: 120–129

21. Nagata S (1999) Biddable death. Nat Cell Biol 1: E143–E145
22. Namura S, Zhu J, Fink K, Endres M, Srinivasan A, Tomaselli KJ, Yuan J, Moskowitz MA (1998) Activation and cleavage of caspase-3 in apoptosis induced by experimental cerebral ischemia. J Neurosci 18: 3659–3668
23. Penninger JM and Kroemer G (2003) Mitochondria, AIF and caspases – rivaling for cell death execution. Nat Cell Biol 5: 97–99
24. Plesnila N, Zhu C, Culmsee C, Gröger M, Moskowitz MA, Blomgren K (2004) Nuclear Translocation of Apoptosis-Inducing Factor (AIF) after Focal Cerebral Ischemia. J Cereb Blood Flow Metab (in press)
25. Plesnila N, Zinkel S, Le DA, Amin-Hanjani S, Wu Y, Qiu J, Chiarugi A, Thomas SS, Kohane DS, Korsmeyer SJ, Moskowitz MA (2001) BID mediates neuronal cell death after oxygen/glucose deprivation and focal cerebral ischemia. Proc Natl Acad Sci USA 98: 15318–15323
26. Robertson GS, Crocker SJ, Nicholson DW, Schulz JB (2000) Neuroprotection by the inhibition of apoptosis. Brain Pathol 10: 283–292
27. Rosenbaum DM, Gupta G, D'Amore J, Singh M, Weidenheim K, Zhang H, Kessler JA (2000) Fas (CD95/APO-1) plays a role in the pathophysiology of focal cerebral ischemia. J Neurosci Res 61: 686–692
28. Scaffidi C, Fulda S, Srinivasan A, Friesen C, Li F, Tomaselli KJ, Debatin KM, Krammer PH, Peter ME (1998) Two CD95 (APO-1/Fas) signaling pathways. EMBO J 17: 1675–1687
29. Schielke GP, Yang GY, Shivers BD, Betz AL (1998) Reduced ischemic brain injury in interleukin-1 beta converting enzyme-deficient mice. J Cereb Blood Flow Metab 18: 180–185
30. Shiga Y, Onodera H, Matsuo Y, Kogure K (1992) Cyclosporin A protects against ischemia-reperfusion injury in the brain. Brain Res 595: 145–148
31. Siesjo BK, Elmer E, Janelidze S, Keep M, Kristian T, Ouyang YB, Uchino H (1999) Role and mechanisms of secondary mitochondrial failure. Acta Neurochir Suppl (Wien) 73: 7–13
32. Springer JE, Azbill RD, Nottingham SA, Kennedy SE (2000) Calcineurin-mediated BAD dephosphorylation activates the caspase-3 apoptotic cascade in traumatic spinal cord injury. J Neurosci 20: 7246–7251
33. Strasser A, O'Connor L, Dixit VM (2000) Apoptosis signaling. Annu Rev Biochem 69: 217–245
34. Susin SA, Lorenzo HK, Zamzami N, Marzo I, Snow BE, Brothers GM, Mangion J, Jacotot E, Costantini P, Loeffler M, Larochette N, Goodlett DR, Aebersold R, Siderovski DP, Penninger JM, Kroemer G (1999) Molecular characterization of mitochondrial apoptosis-inducing factor. Nature 397: 441–446
35. Susin SA, Lorenzo HK, Zamzami N, Marzo I, Snow BE, Brothers GM, Mangion J, Jacotot E, Costantini P, Loeffler M, Larochette N, Goodlett DR, Aebersold R, Siderovski DP, Penninger JM, Kroemer G (1999) Molecular characterization of mitochondrial apoptosis-inducing factor. Nature 397: 441–446
36. Velier JJ, Ellison JA, Kikly KK, Spera PA, Barone FC, Feuerstein GZ (1999) Caspase-8 and caspase-3 are expressed by different populations of cortical neurons undergoing delayed cell death after focal stroke in the rat. J Neurosci 19: 5932–5941
37. Wang K, Yin XM, Chao DT, Milliman CL, Korsmeyer SJ (1996) BID: a novel BH3 domain-only death agonist. Genes Dev 10: 2859–2869
38. Wei MC, Lindsten T, Mootha VK, Weiler S, Gross A, Ashiya M, Thompson CB, Korsmeyer SJ (2000) tBID, a membrane-targeted death ligand, oligomerizes BAK to release cytochrome c. Genes Dev 14: 2060–2071
39. Yan C, Chen J, Chen D, Minami M, Pei W, Yin XM, Simon RP (2000) Overexpression of the cell death suppressor Bcl-w in ischemic brain: implications for a neuroprotective role via the mitochondrial pathway. J Cereb Blood Flow Metab 20: 620–630
40. Yin XM, Wang K, Gross A, Zhao Y, Zinkel S, Klocke B, Roth KA, Korsmeyer SJ (1999) Bid-deficient mice are resistant to Fas-induced hepatocellular apoptosis. Nature 400: 886–891
41. Yoshimoto T and Siesjo BK (1999) Posttreatment with the immunosuppressant cyclosporin A in transient focal ischemia. Brain Res 839: 283–291
42. Yuan J and Yankner BA (2000) Apoptosis in the nervous system. Nature 407: 802–809
43. Zha J, Weiler S, Oh KJ, Wei MC, Korsmeyer SJ (2000) Posttranslational N-Myristoylation of BID as a Molecular Switch for Targeting Mitochondria and Apoptosis. Science 290: 1761–1765
44. Zou H, Li Y, Liu X, Wang X (1999) An APAF-1 cytochrome c multimeric complex is a functional apoptosome that activates procaspase-9. J Biol Chem 274: 11549–11556

Correspondence: Nikolaus Plesnila, M.D., University of Munich, Institute for Surgical Research, Marchioninistr. 27, 81377 Munchen, Germany. e-mail: plesnila@icf.med.uni-muenchen.de

Acta Neurochir (2004) [Suppl] 89: 21–35

Printed in Austria

Signalling mechanisms for survival of lesioned motoneurons

S. Wiese, M. Beck, C. Karch, and **M. Sendtner**

Institute for Clinical Neurobiology, Würzburg, Germany

Summary

Mechanisms controlling neuronal survival play an important role both during development and after birth, in particular when the nervous system is lesioned. Isolated embryonic motoneurons and other types of primary neurons have been a useful tool for studying basic mechanisms underlying neuronal cell death during development and under pathophysiological conditions after neurotrauma. These studies have led to the identification of neurotrophic factors which under physiological conditions regulate survival and functional properties, and after neurotrauma promote regeneration and plasticity. Functional analysis of these molecules, in particular by generation of gene knockout mice, has led to a more detailed understanding of complex requirements of individual types of neurons for their survival and also paved the way for a better understanding of the signalling pathways in lesioned neurons which decide on cell death or survival after axotomy and other pathophysiological conditions. These findings could ultimately lead to a rational basis for therapeutic approaches aiming at improving neuronal survival and regeneration after neurotrauma.

Keywords: Neuronal survival; neuronal death; neurotrophic factors; gene knock-out mice.

Developmental motoneuron cell death as a model for studying signalling pathways for neuronal survival

Pioneer work by Viktor Hamburger and others during the first part of the 20th century have shown that the developmental cell death of motoneurons is guided by influences provided from their target tissue [45, 46]. Removal of limb buds in developing chick embryos massively enhances the extent of motoneuron cell death, and transplantation of an additional limb reduces the number of dying motoneurons. Thus, the individual organism can react to deviations from genetically determined developmental programs, and this kind of plasticity might have contributed to the generation of a highly complex nervous system in higher vertebrates during evolution. The model that skeletal muscle plays a major role in regulating motoneuron survival during development has been recently challenged by the observation that mice deficient for erb-B3, the receptor for glial growth factor (GGF), show a severe deficit of developing Schwann cells, and then, as a consequence, a significant reduction (79%) in motoneurons [87]. Thus developing Schwann cells are at least as important for motoneurons as skeletal muscle. However, these data could also indicate that motoneurons first become dependent on muscle-derived neurotrophic support and then, subsequently, on Schwann cell-derived factors. Indeed, when skeletal muscle is destroyed during embryonic development by a cre/loxP-mediated strategy [44], motoneuron survival in the lumbar spinal cord is highly diminished, as expected from the early data obtained from experiments in chick when limb buds are removed [81]. In conclusion, it has to be assumed that neurotrophic factors from various sources play together in regulating survival and functional integrity of motoneurons. This scenario appears even more complex with respect to early findings that motoneuron cell death in vertebrates can also occur in a target-independent manner. Rita Levi-Montalcini and others have shown [55, 77, 82] that during early development of the chick embryo around day 4, massive cell death can be observed in a specific population of motoneurons in the ventral cervical spinal cord. This type of cell death is highly synchronized, in contrast to motoneuron cell death observed in this and other regions of the developing chick spinal cord between embryonic day 6 to 10, which roughly corresponds to embryonic day 14 to postnatal day 3 in the mouse or rat. A recent study [113] has shown that this type of early motoneuron cell death occurs in a target-independent manner and may be determined by a cell-autonomous program. Taken together, these data suggest that cell death programs in motoneurons probably change during development, and at least some of the motoneurons pass through an early phase when cell-autonomous and/or target-independent processes regulate cell death and then undergo a phase when signals from skeletal muscle play a major role. Subsequently, signals from Schwann cells such as CNTF and other survival factors acting through signalling pathways involving Stat-3 contribute to the maintenance of motoneurons, and arising evidence from experiments with various mouse mutants suggests that postnatal survival of motoneurons becomes increasingly dependent again on cell autonomous processes such as sufficient expression of the "survival of motoneuron" (SMN) protein [50, 70] and protection from glutamate-mediated toxicity [90]. Further research has to show how these signals and the intracellular signaling pathways play together and how the motoneurons react to disturbances of individual signals. The availability of mouse mutants in which individual signals are disrupted either by classical homologous recombination or in a cell type-specific or otherwise inducible manner by use of the Cre/loxP and other recombination techniques will help to understand such processes and thus could provide a basis for strategies aiming at improvement of motoneuron survival after trauma.

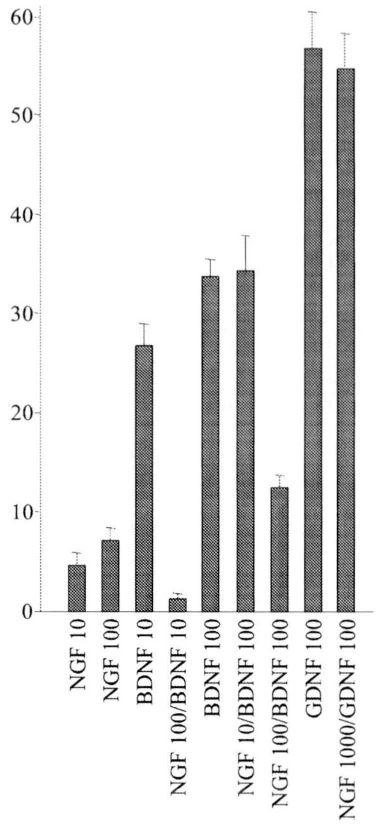

Fig. 1. NGF antagonizes BDNF-mediated survival of mouse motoneurons in culture. Motoneurons were isolated from lumbar spinal cord of 14 day old mouse embryos [109]. Survival of motoneurons was determined by counting surviving motoneurons after 3 days in culture. Values shown are % of initially plated neurons in the culture dish. BDNF and NGF were added at concentrations indicated at 10 or 100 pg/ml. The survival effect of BDNF is significantly reduced in the presence of NGF at equimolar concentrations, and completely abolished when NGF is given at doses 10 times higher than BDNF. Note that maximal concentration of NGF in this experiment was 100 pg/ml, which is below the concentration thought to saturate low-affinity neurotrophin receptors. NGF could not reduce the survival response initiated by GDNF, even when the concentration was increased to a level of 1000 pg/ml, thus suggesting that NGF acts as a specific antagonist, probably at the receptor level, rather than acting as an independent cell death effector on these cultured motoneurons

Neurotrophic factors for motoneurons

Nerve growth factor (NGF) was the first neurotrophic factor which has been discovered. Most models on how neurotrophic factors act are still based on findings with NGF. It is a prototypic target-derived neurotrophic molecule that, among other neuronal cell types, regulates survival of subpopulations of sensory paravertebral sympathetic neurons. In the meantime, more than a dozen additional neurotrophic factors have been identified and characterized on a molecular level. This list includes neurotrophins which are related to NGF [9]. At least 3 neurotrophins, brain-derived neurotrophic factor, neurotrophin-3 and neurotrophin-4, but not NGF, support motoneuron survival [47, 49, 96].

Motoneurons are also supported by other families of neurotrophic molecules. Some of these molecules are only expressed postnatally, indicating that the requirement of motoneurons for these factors changes during development, and that postnatal survival is also controlled by neurotrophic factors. Moreover, it is very likely that these factors influence specific properties of motoneurons such as the regulation of transmitter synthesis and release, axon outgrowth and dendrite arborization as well as synaptic stability (reviewed in [94]). It is therefore not surprising that individual factors have not been identified so far that serve prototypic functions, i.e. the control of survival during the period of physiological motoneuron cell death.

The CNTF family supports motoneuron survival through activation of complex membrane receptors involving gp130 and LIFR-β [73]. Factors which

Table 1. *Neurotrophic factors for motoneurons and their receptors*

	Receptor on motoneurons
1. Neurotrophins	
Brain-derived neurotrophic factor (BDNF)	$p75^{NTR}$, trk-B
Neurotrophin-3 (NT-3)	$p75^{NTR}$, trk-C
Neurotrophin-4/5 (NT-4/5)	$p75^{NTR}$, trk-B
2. CNTF/LIF family	
Ciliary neurotrophic factor (CNTF)	CNTFRα, LIFRβ, gp130
Leukemia inhibitory factor (LIF)	LIFRβ, gp130
Cardiotrophin-1 (CT-1)	?, LIFRβ, gp130
Cardiotrophin-1 like cytokine (CLC)	CNTFRα?, LIFRβ, gp130
3. Hepatocyte growth factor/Scatter factor	
(HGF/SF)	c-met
4. Insulin-like growth factors	
IGF-I	IGFR-1
IGF-II	IGFR-1, Mannose-6P receptor
5. Glial-derived neurotrophic factor and related factors	
Glial-derived neurotrophic factor (GDNF)	GFRα1, c-ret
Neurturin (NTR)	GFRα2, c-ret
Persephin	GFRα4, c-ret
Artemin	GFRα3, c-ret

bind to such complexes are ciliary neurotrophic factor [4], leukemia-inhibitory factor [49], cardiotrophin-1 (Pennica *et al.* 1995) and the recently identified cardiotrophin-like cytokine (CLC) [84, 93, 97] which also can bind to the CNTF receptor complex [32].

Motoneuron survival in culture is also supported by members of the glial-derived neurotrophic factor (GDNF) gene family of transforming growth factor-β-related survival factors [48, 118]. Factors which support motoneuron survival include GDNF [48], neurturin [52], persephin [66], and artemin [6]. These molecules act through receptors involving the c-ret tyrosine kinase, and specific α-receptors [5].

HGF is a heterodimeric protein which supports motoneuron survival [30, 74, 114]. Interestingly, only lumbar motoneurons from 5 day old chick embryos survive with HGF, but not motoneurons from thoracic or cervical spinal cord [76]. The c-met tyrosine kinase is expressed in lumbar but not in thoracic motoneurons between embryonic day 5 and 10 during the period of physiological motoneuron cell death in chick. However, the expression of c-met in lumbar motoneurons seems to be regulated by other target tissue-derived factors than HGF. This conclusion is based on the observation that the massive cell death of motoneurons which occurs in the lumbar spinal cord after limb bud removal cannot be reduced by treatment with HGF, probably because the c-met receptor is down-regulated by limb-bud removal and signals which lead to expression of this receptor are thus removed. Thus, HGF is an example of a neurotrophic factor which influences survival only of subpopulations of motoneurons, and needs cooperation with other signals in order to exert its survival-promoting effect under physiological conditions. The list of molecules that support motoneuron survival is still growing, and it can be expected to become even longer during the next few years.

Motoneurons are also supported by insulin-like growth factor-1 (IGF-1) and IGF-2 [4]. In cultures of isolated embryonic chick spinal motoneurons, the survival-promoting effects of IGFs are relatively low, in contrast to cultures of embryonic rat motoneurons which can be maintained in serum-free medium [49]. However, when IGFs are combined with other neurotrophic factors such as CNTF, this leads to supra-additive survival effects [4]. This was one of the first demonstrations that neurotrophic factors potentiate each other in supporting motoneuron survival, suggesting that survival of motoneurons in vivo depends on a complex cooperation of more than one factor.

Similarly, when BDNF was administered for prolonged periods to lesioned facial motoneurons via a gene therapy approach, it supported survival but could not prevent atrophy of the neuronal cell bodies [41]. Only when BDNF and CNTF were added together, a significant anti-atrophic effect was observed. Thus motoneurons may depend on more than one neurotrophic factor, and development, survival and proper function of these cells could be modulated by such factors in a way where they have to play together in a well-balanced manner.

This observation is important for the design of therapeutic strategies with neurotrophic factors. It predicts that the administration of a single factor will not meet the physiological requirements of motoneurons, especially in a situation where these cells are deprived from their target over prolonged periods and should be stimulated to regrow their axons over long distances.

Signaling pathways for neurotrophic factor mediated motoneuron survival

The neurotrophins have served as a prototypic gene family to define the signaling pathways which regulate survival and other effects in primary neurons [92]. A significant contribution to this research was provided by investigations employing the rat PC 12 pheochromocytoma cell line. Signaling through neurotrophin receptors which include members of the trk gene family, involves several pathways. Initiation depends on the cytosolic adaptor protein Shc, the activation of PLC-γ and the PI-3-kinase/AKT-pathways directly at the level of the trk transmembrane tyrosine kinases.

The Shc adapter proteins have been focus of research, as they can couple trk-signaling to the Ras/MAP-kinase pathway, which is involved in promoting neuronal survival and neurite outgrowth. Experiments with PC-12 cells [8] and with primary sympathetic neurons [11] have shown that activated Ras can support differentiation and survival of neuronal cells. At least in PC-12 cells, sustained activation of the MAPK pathway [1, 102, 111] can promote differentiation versus mitogenic effects of NGF in comparison to epidermal growth factor (EGF). It has been suggested that sustained activation of the MAPK pathway is also responsible for the neurotrophin-mediated survival effect in neuronal cell lines and primary neurons. Recently, a second Ras-independent pathway for activation of the MAPK pathway has been shown to be involved in NGF-mediated differentiation [117]. This brings activation mechanisms upstream from Ras and other GTPases into focus which transduce the signal from receptor molecules to the MAPK and other pathways.

In neurons several forms of Shc exist, named ShcA, ShcB, and ShcC/N-shc [16]. Expression of these isoforms is strictly controlled during development. Only little is known so far whether differences in their expression influence signal transduction downstream of trk receptors, e.g. by determining targets involved in mediating cellular effects of neurotrophic factors including the survival of specific neuronal cell types at specific developmental stages. The ratio of ShcA and ShcC/N-Shc expression deserves particular attention. ShcC/N-Shc has been detected as a neuron-specific Shc isoform [72], which mediates the coupling of trk signaling to Ras activation. Whereas ShcA is expressed ubiquitously, ShcC expression is only found in the nervous system. Interestingly, the upregulation of ShcC corresponds to a downregulation of ShcA expression in the brain at a developmental stage when neuronal cells become postmitotic [18]. Intriguingly at least some populations of neurons including motoneurons become dependent on neurotrophic factors for their survival at the same time. It is tempting to speculate that this switch from ShcA to ShcC expression might be responsible for converting the neurotrophic factor-mediated signal from differentiation to survival [92]. The Shc binding site in trk-B has been mutated in mice [68], indicating that differences between various neurotrophic factors exist in the utilization of this pathway for mediating survival and neurite outgrowth effects. Under these conditions, NT-4-mediated survival effects were more dramatically reduced than BDNF-dependent differentiation or survival. Complete loss of the NT-4-dependent D-hair sensory cells but no change in BDNF-dependent slowly adapting mechanotransducing sensory neurons was observed. Motoneuron survival has not been investigated in these mice so far, and it remains to be demonstrated whether motoneuron function, survival and regeneration is are altered when the Shc binding site is mutated in the trkB receptor.

Besides the Ras/MAPK pathway, a second pathway involving activation of PI-3K seems to be highly important for neuronal survival [29]. Direct association of PI-3K with trk receptors has been found under specific experimental conditions [79]. However, it is now widely accepted that Shc signaling plays a major role in activation of PI-3K downstream of trks in neuronal cells [10, 19, 42]. The PI-3-kinase in turn leads to activation of Akt, a serine/threonine kinase with a broad spectrum of substrates including the proapoptotic Bad [19], caspase-9 [14], the forkhead transcription factor FKHRL1 [13] and IKKα kinase, leading to activation of the NFκB pathway [83, 89]. It remains to be seen which of these downstream pathways is responsible for neuronal survival, in particular under pathophysiological conditions when axons are lesioned.

A third important pathway, in particular for motoneuron survival is the activation of PLCγ1 [78, 92, 101]. This pathway leads to increased release of free Ca^{2+} from intracellular stores, which in turn can activate cyclic AMP response-element–binding protein (CREB) [36]. In addition, elevated intracellular Ca^{2+} levels also activate the small GTP-binding protein Rap1 but not Ras [43]. This leads to activation of B-Raf but not to activation of Raf-1. In developing motoneurons, B-Raf is expressed at relatively high levels during the period of physiological cell death [110]. Thus a link between various pathways exists, and increased levels of Ca^{2+} could contribute to activation of Rafs, which seem to play a central role both in activation of the MAPK pathway and also as effector kinases for bcl-2 which phosphorylate BAD and thus inhibit its proapoptotic activity [106, 107].

Dysregulation of these mechanisms might also contribute to the pathophysiology of motoneuron atrophy after nerve lesion. Future studies have to show for example which members of the Shc family are expressed in motoneurons after lesion, whether expression changes during prolonged time periods without contact to target tissues, and how these mechanisms then influence axon regrowth. Together with the elucidation of signals from glial cells and extracellular matrix which stimulate axon growth, these data could provide a basis for development of rational therapy for regeneration of motor axons to denervated skeletal muscle.

cAMP and motoneuron survival

Elevation of cyclic AMP (cAMP) can provide a survival signal for motoneurons even in the absence of neurotrophic factors [63]. This could be of high physiological relevance, as many neurotransmitters act via G-protein coupled receptors, and thus change cAMP levels in motoneurons. In the absence of neurotrophic factors, cAMP only promotes short-term survival of spinal motoneurons in culture when merosin is used as a substrate. However, under these specific conditions, the combination of elevation of intracellular cAMP and neurotrophic factors leads to prolonged survival of motoneurons over periods exceeding 3 weeks. Similarly, elevation of cAMP levels has also been shown to increase survival of superior cervical ganglion neuron and cerebellar granule cells. These cAMP-mediated survival effects seem to be independent from PI-3K-activation, since inhibitors such as Wortmannin could not abolish the pro-survival effects of cAMP. A first indication how these survival pathways could be linked was given by the demonstration that cAMP elevation can increase the recruitment of the trk-B-receptor to the plasma membrane in retinal ganglion cells (Meyer-Franke *et al.* 1998). This mechanism could be highly relevant for the development of therapeutic strategies implying neurotrophic factors. Studies with primary neurons in cell culture have shown that BDNF exposure leads to a rapid downregulation of the cell membrane exposure of trk-B [15], and therapeutic administration of BDNF at high concentrations to axotomized motoneurons after facial nerve transection only leads to transient rescue effects [104], even when BDNF is administered chronically with osmotic pumps or repeatedly by systemic injections. Thus inhibition of transfer of trk-B from intracellular to cell membrane compartments could play a role in the downregulation of trk-B survival signals under such conditions.

The effect of elevated cAMP on motoneuron survival is strongest when the motoneurons are cultured on merosin [63], a synapse-specific isoform of laminin. When motoneurons from 15 day old rat or 14 day old mouse embryos are cultured on a laminin substrate (S. Wiese and M. Sendtner, unpublished observations), the survival effect of elevated cAMP is much weaker. Thus, an important question for further research is whether merosin and laminin differentially influence the rise of free Ca^{2+} after cAMP stimulation. This may also be of importance for the elucidation of other specific effects of neurotrophic factors beyond support of survival, such as axon outgrowth, synaptic stability and fine tuning of synapse activity.

Recently, we could show that B-Raf but not C-Raf is involved in mediating survival responses of neurotrophic factors in motoneurons [110]. These serine/threonine kinases associate with ras and play a crucial role in the downstream propagation of the neurotrophic signals to the MAPK and the PI3-K/Akt pathways [111]. C-Raf activity is inhibited by cAMP elevation in various types of cells including neurons. In contrast B-Raf is activated by cAMP and thus signals from neurotransmitter receptors and neurotrophic factor receptors might come together at the level of this specific kinase [33].

These data also suggest that neurotrophic factors should not be considered as the only players which regulate motoneuron cell death under physiological conditions. Indeed, motoneuron survival in culture in the presence of neurotrophic factors strongly depends on the presence of components of the extracellular matrix. Laminin was one of the first molecules which was found to potentiate the survival effect of neurotrophic factors [31]. When motoneurons from 6 day old chick embryos are isolated and cultured in the presence of laminin, about 55% of these isolated motoneurons can be maintained for periods longer than 1 week [4] with CNTF. However, this survival effect significantly drops when the concentration of laminin used to coat the culture dishes is reduced from 10 to 1 $\mu g ml^{-1}$ (Table 2). In the absence of laminin, the survival effect of CNTF even drops to 3.7% which is not statistically different from control when motoneurons are cultured in the absence of neurotrophic factors (2.4% survival). These data indicate that integrin signaling cooperates with neurotrophic factors

Table 2. *Influence of laminin on CNTF-mediated survival of isolated embryonic chick motoneurons*

Neurotrophic factor	Amount of laminin used for culture dish coating (μg)	Survival of motoneurons after 3 days in culture (% of originally plated cells)
CNTF	10	55.4
FGF-2	10	44.4
CNTF+FGF-2	10	95.8
None	10	2.4
CNTF	1	22.5
FGF-2	1	22.4
CNTF+FGF-2	1	53.3
None	1	0.0
CNTF	–	3.7
FGF-2	–	8.9
CNTF+FGF-2	–	12.5
None	–	0.0

Reproduced with permission from [95].

in mediating motoneuron survival, and it will be interesting to see whether integrin signaling influences cAMP levels in motoneurons and thus plays together with neurotrophic factors in regulating specific functions in motoneurons.

The role of neuronal activity and glutamate for motoneuron survival

In many types of neurons, removal of afferent input leads to increased cell death in vivo [80]. This corresponds to observations that neurons can be maintained in cell culture under conditions which mimic depolarization such as elevated potassium concentration [105] or even addition of glutamate receptor agonists at optimal concentrations [64]. However, various populations of neurons differ in their capacity to survive in culture in the presence of increased levels of potassium or glutamate. Whereas 35 mM K^+ in the culture medium can support survival of sympathetic neurons derived from 10 day old chick embryos [105], motoneurons from 5 or 6 day old chick embryos cannot survive for periods longer than 3 days under the same culture conditions. In this respect, motoneurons show similar behavior as retinal ganglion cells, which also do not survive when the potassium concentration in the culture medium is elevated [64]. Contrarily, survival with the neurotrophic factor BDNF was strongly enhanced in isolated retinal ganglion cells when the cells were depolarized or even when NMDA or kainic acid were added to these cultures. The effect could be mediated by elevation of cAMP, as inhibitors of protein kinase A could prevent the potentiation of the BDNF survival effect by increased potassium or glutamate agonists in the culture medium. These data also suggest that intracellular Ca^{2+} elevation is responsible for this effect.

Glutamate toxicity is considered as a major pathomechanism after neurotrauma. Embryonic motoneurons express NMDA receptors [51] and AMPA receptors including subtypes of AMPA receptors which mediate Ca^{2+} influx in response to glutamate [60]. When these motoneurons are exposed to elevated concentrations of glutamate or NMDA in vitro, motoneuron cell death is not enhanced [61]. This seems surprising with respect to the observation that massive cell death occurs under the same conditions in cultures of cortical neurons (M.S., unpublished observations). Even when the motoneurons are depolarized in order to remove the Mg^{2+}-block of NMDA receptors, this does not influence motoneuron survival in cell culture, suggesting that isolated embryonic motoneurons are quite resistant to glutamate toxicity. On the other side, NMDA or glutamate exposure does not potentiate the survival effect of BDNF or other neurotrophic factors, as observed with isolated retinal ganglion cells [64]. Despite this negative effect, motoneurons show specific responses to enhanced glutamate in the culture medium. Glutamate treatment leads to specific inhibition of dendrite growth in a fully reversible manner. Axon outgrowth was not affected under the same culture conditions, suggesting that glutamate could play an important role in plasticity of dendrite growth and synapse formation between motoneurons and other types of neurons within the spinal cord.

Intracellular signals for neuronal survival: the role of members of the IAP family

Not very much is known about the downstream signals involved in execution of motoneuron cell death cell and neurotrophic factor-mediated survival. Research on the role bcl-2 has guided the way to our present knowledge. Overexpression of bcl-2 significantly reduces motoneuron cell death during development [28, 58]. However, mice in which bcl-2 expression is abolished by homologous recombination show only a small reduction of motoneuron numbers at birth [65], indicating either that bcl-2-related molecules can substitute for this deficiency or that bcl-2 and related molecules are not physiologically necessary for motoneuron survival during development. Interestingly, motoneuron cell death in bcl-2 −/− mice is enhanced only during the postnatal period, leading to loss of around 40% of facial motoneurons in 6 week old mice. This suggests that bcl-2 becomes important for postnatal survival at least of subpopulations of motoneurons. However, bcl-2 deficient motoneurons do not lose their responsiveness to neurotrophic factors. BDNF and CNTF are still capable of rescuing motoneurons from lesion-induced cell death after facial nerve transection in newborn animals. Nevertheless, survival in response to these neurotrophic factors was lower in bcl-2 deficient mice indicating that subpopulations depend on bcl-2 for survival after nerve lesion, and/or that compensation by other antiapoptotic members of the bcl-2 family is only incomplete.

Neurons from BAX-deficient mice [22, 53] are resistant against cell death after neurotrophic factor deprivation. This observation provides a second indication that members of the bcl-2 family are involved, and that mitochondria play a role in motoneuron cell death. Recently, it has been shown that BAX-dependent release of cytochrome c from mitochondria plays an essential role in the initiation of cell death in NGF-deprived sympathetic neurons [23]. However, microinjection of cytochrome c into the cytoplasm could not initiate cell death when the primary sympathetic neurons were grown in the presence of NGF. Based on these observations, it was speculated that NGF leads to a rapid production of an intracellular protein, which protects cells from proapoptotic actions of cytochrome c [75]. Furthermore, it was concluded that such protective molecules are expressed at low basal levels and upregulated within short time after NGF exposure.

Members of the IAP/ITA family are candidates for such protective proteins. They inhibit the activation of procaspase-9 [24], which is initiated by cytochrome c and Apaf-1 [98, 99]. Furthermore, they inhibit the function of activated caspase-3, -6 and -7, and thus at least at two levels interfere with cellular programs for apoptosis [25, 91]. The identification and cloning of the chick *ita* gene [26], which encodes a protein of 611 amino acids with highest homology to the human cIAP-2 gene (also called HIAP-1 or MIHC), allowed us to investigate the involvement of this protein in NGF-mediated survival of developing chick sympathetic and sensory neurons. We could show that NGF rapidly induced ITA expression in cultured sympathetic and sensory neurons (Fig. 2). This upregulation of ITA mRNA and protein levels involves the PI-3K pathway. Overexpression of ITA in primary sensory and sympathetic neurons can promote neuronal survival in the absence of NGF, and antisense expression of ITA can abolish the NGF survival effect in sensory and sympathetic neurons. These actions are apparently mediated through the baculovirus IAP repeat (BIR domains) of the ITA protein, as expression of a BIR-deleted form of ITA was without any effect on neuronal survival.

These data suggest that members of the IAP family which include the mammalian IAP-2 and XIAP are important molecules involved in the signaling machinery for neurotrophic factor-mediated survival of sympathetic and sensory neurons. The expression of inhibitors for caspases could be an essential mechanism which contributes to motoneuron survival once these caspases are activated (Fig. 3), and they probably could be of high importance in protecting motoneurons against any kind of proapoptotic signaling which might occur during postnatal life and which has to be neutralized for further maintenance of these cells.

A role for cell death signalling in axotomized motoneurons?

Cell autonomous mechanisms play an important role in deciding on survival or cell death during development of lower organisms such as C. elegans. The ces-2 gene which triggers programmed cell death [62] is expressed specifically in two distinct pharyngeal motoneurons in the worm and initiates death in these specific cells. Such cell-autonomous cell death genes have not been identified so far in motoneurons from higher vertebrates. Nethertheless, active cell death mechanisms play a role during an early phase of development when motoneuron cell death apparently occurs in a target-independent manner. The cell death receptor Fas and the corresponding Fas ligand are expressed in early motoneurons, and Fas has been found to transmit a cell death signal in cultured motoneurons from 12.5 day old mouse embryos [86]. Fas and Fas-ligand are expressed early during development in motoneurons, and it has been suggested that the coexpression of these two molecules in principle allows cell-autonomous cell death programs. When embryonic motoneurons were cultured for 3 days with neurotrophic factors, they became resistant to Fas-induced cell death, either by interference with downstream-effectors such as the activated caspase-8 and caspase-3,

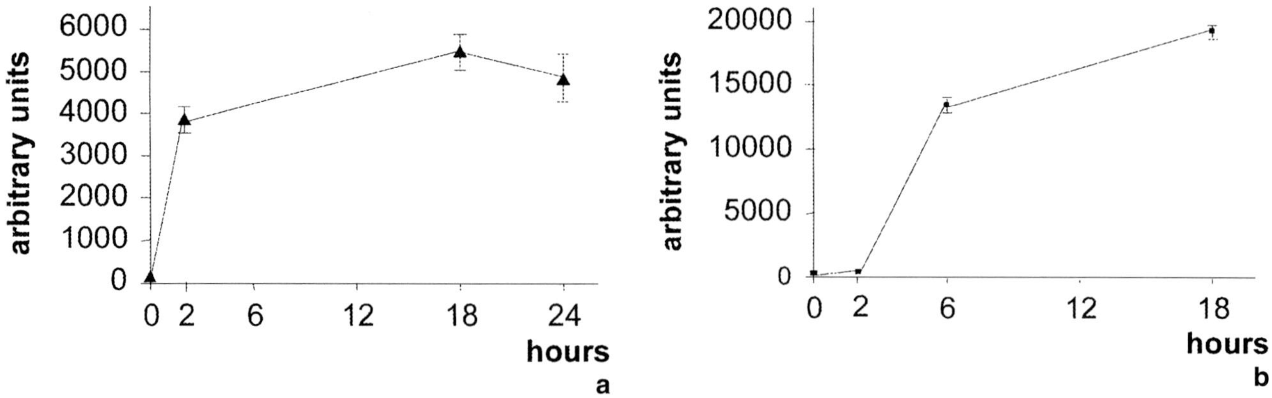

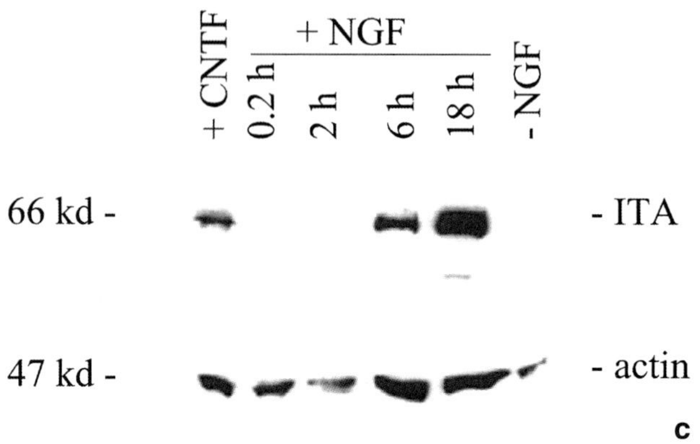

Fig. 2. NGF and CNTF promote upregulation of the avian inhibitor of T-cell apoptosis *(ITA)* protein, a homologue of mammalian IAPs in cultured sensory and sympathetic neurons. IAPs are potent inhibitors of caspases, and thus could participate in the survival response of neurons to neurotrophic factors. See [108] for details. Reproduced with permission from this publication. –▲– sensory neurons; –■– sympathetic neurons

or by allowing motoneurons to mature to a stage when they are resistant to cell-autonomous cell death programs, or by both mechanisms. Thus, Fas and Fas-ligand could promote motoneuron cell death when these cells do not yet depend on or even cannot react to neurotrophic factors, and further studies for example involving Bid-deficient mice which are resistant to Fas-induced cell death could be of great help to understand the physiological role of Fas-mediated cell death for motoneurons.

The p75 neurotrophin receptor ($p75^{NTR}$) shares structural and functional similarities with other transmembrane molecules of the Fas/Apo-1/CD95 and tumor necrosis factor receptor −1 family (see [71] for review). This receptor is expressed at high levels in developing motoneurons, then disappears, but is highly reexpressed after nerve lesion. In a variety of cellular contexts in vitro and in vivo, $p75^{NTR}$ mediates cell death after binding of NGF, in particular when trk receptors are not expressed [17, 40]. Injection of neutralizing antibodies into the eye of early chick embryos has shown that NGF and $p75^{NTR}$ are involved in mediating early cell death of retinal ganglion cells which have just been formed and are starting to grow axons [37, 39]. In this respect, NGF and $p75^{NTR}$ are involved in an early phase of cell death which is not regulated by the target-tissue. In this specific case, the source of NGF were microglial cells which had invaded the retina during these early developmental stages [39].

The role of $p75^{NTR}$ as a mediator of cell death has also been shown in basal forebrain cholinergic neurons [116]. Overexpression of the cytoplasmic part of the $p75^{NTR}$ in mice [57] leads to significant losses of several populations of neurons including motoneurons in the facial nucleus. Thus, it appears intriguing that $p75^{NTR}$ could have similar functions in motoneurons, in particular when this receptor is expressed at high levels after axotomy. Indeed, when the expression of this receptor was abolished in adult $p75^{NTR}$ −/− mice, survival and regeneration of axotomized motoneurons was improved in comparison to control animals [35], and overexpression of the cytoplasmic part of $p75^{NTR}$ enhanced lesion-induced cell death of facial motoneurons in adult mice [57]. Moreover, application of NGF to axotomized sciatic [69] or facial [96] motoneurons significantly increased the rate of cell death in rats or mice [109]. These results are compatible with the assumption that $p75^{NTR}$ is a cell death receptor in developing motoneurons. On the other side and in contrast to other neuronal populations [7, 103, 115],

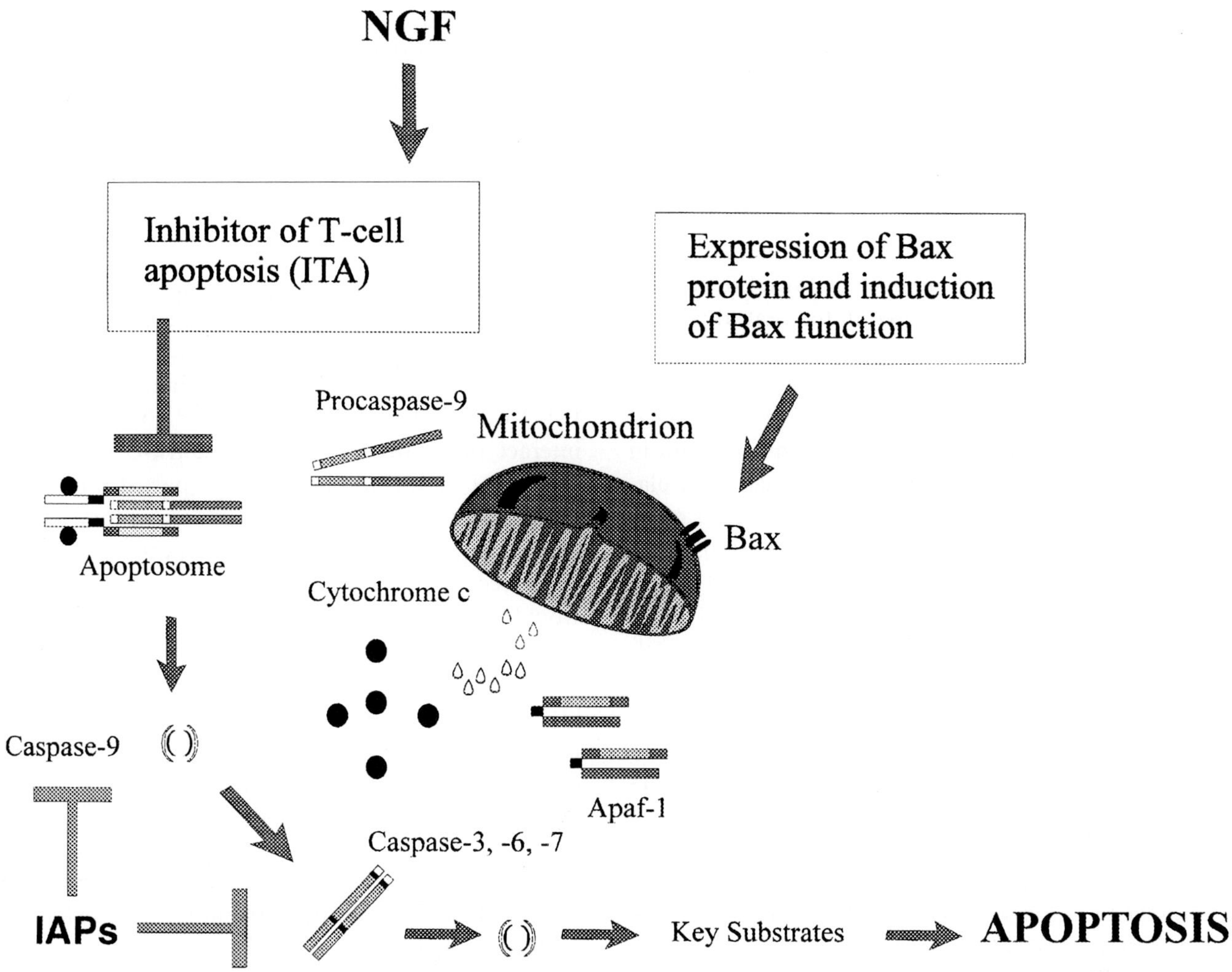

Fig. 3. Signaling pathways for neurotrophic factor mediated survival of motoneurons. Recent studies [23] have shown that injection of cytochrome-C into the cytoplasm of cultured neurons can induce apoptosis only when nerve growth factor is absent or added after the injection of cytochrome-C. This has lead to the conclusion that nerve growth factor and other neurotrophic factors lead to upregulation of an activity which directly interferes with the activation of apoptosome activity and downstream caspases. In the absence of neurotrophic factors, cytochrome-C is released from mitochondria by a process in which Bax is involved. This leads to the formation of apoptosomes by a process also requiring Apaf-1 and ATP. By this means, procaspase-9 is cleaved and activated. Caspase-9 in turn can cleave procaspase-3, -6 and/or -7, which then activate downstream substrates, among them ICAD (inhibitor of caspase-activated Dnase *(CAD)*) and finally leads to apoptosis of the neuron. Members of the IAP-family (inhibitor of apoptosis protein) can block activated caspases and inhibit these regulatory steps in the execution of apoptosis. In cultured sensory and sympathetic neurons, NGF and CNTF upregulate ITA expression at least 20 fold. This upregulation takes place within less than 6 hours. Thus, ITA and mammalian homologues of this protein could be essential mediators in the downstream signaling machinery for neurotrophic factor-mediated survival of primary neurons

the number of motoneurons in 6–9 week old $p75^{NTR}$ −/− mice is reduced in comparison to wild-type mice, as revealed by quantification of facial motoneurons and axon profiles in brain stem and peripheral nerves [35, 109]. However, in the case of basal forebrain cholinergic neurons, contradictory results have been obtained in the meantime so that at least one of the originally published reports apparently is not reproducible, and the findings thus do not support a proapoptotic function through the p75 neurotrophin receptor in postnatal basal forebrain cholinergic neurons [103].

Motoneurons do not only express high levels of $p75^{NTR}$ after axotomy, but also under physiological conditions during early development. Expression of this receptor molecule apparently occurs before the motoneurons have gained contact with skeletal muscle and before these motoneurons become responsive at least to BDNF for their survival. In order to test the possibility that NGF and p75^{NTR} are mediators of the early phase of motoneuron cell death in brachial spinal cord, Frade and Barde have investigated cell death in the spinal cord of p75^{NTR} −/− and NGF −/− mice between E10.5–12.5, before the period of classical target-dependent cell death starts [38]. In such animals, an increase in the thickness of the mantel zone was observed. However, the number of ISLET-1 positive motoneurons was not increased in the ventral portion of the spinal cord of these mutant mice.

In order to test the role of p75^{NTR} and the actions of NGF on developing motoneurons during the classical period of target-dependent motoneuron cell death in more detail, we have developed techniques for isolation of motoneurons from lumbar spinal cord of 14 day old wildtype and p75^{NTR} −/− mice [109]. NGF did not support long-term survival of isolated mouse motoneurons. In contrary, it reduced the survival effects of BDNF and NT-3 in wildtype but not p75^{NTR} −/− motoneurons. On a first aspect, these data favor the model of p75^{NTR} as a cell death receptor on motoneurons. However, the quantities of NGF which interfered with the survival responses of BDNF and NT-3 were very low (7×10^{-13} M) (Fig. 1). They did not reach the levels necessary for saturating those low-affinity binding sites on primary neurons which are thought to correspond to p75^{NTR} receptors [59, 88]. Recently, it has been described that p75^{NTR} can be expressed in neuronal cells in a conformation conferring high-affinity binding of NT-3 [21]. However, under the same experimental conditions NGF did not bind to p75^{NTR} when added at 10^{-12} M.

Observations that very low quantities of NGF interfere with BDNF and NT-3 effects in neurons could be explained by a model in which the p75^{NTR} is part of the high-affinity receptor for BDNF and probably also NT-3. Previous observations that NGF enhances motoneuron survival at later developmental stages in chick [85] when p75^{NTR} expression is low [34] suggest that the presence of p75^{NTR} could enhance the specificity of BDNF and NT-3. Determination of motoneuron cell numbers in newborn NGF −/− mice or 1 week old NGF +/− mice after facial nerve lesion at birth could help to further define whether endogenous NGF interferes at neurotrophin receptors in developing and/or postnatal lesioned motoneurons. Such experiments are underway in several labs.

Reduction of NT-3- and BDNF-mediated survival by NGF is not seen in p75^{NTR} −/− motoneurons. This observation also suggests that p75^{NTR} receptors are components of the high-affinity binding sites for NT-3 and BDNF on E14 lumbar motoneurons and do not constitute separate NGF receptors. We have also observed that the BDNF dose necessary for half-maximal survival is shifted from 1.2×10^{-12} M in wildtype motoneurons to 5.4×10^{-12} M in p75^{NTR} −/− motoneurons. This supports previous data that trk homodimers are not equivalent to high-affinity neurotrophin receptors in primary neurons [56, 112]. Our data suggest that p75^{NTR} is part of the high-affinity receptor complex for BDNF and possibly also NT-3 on motoneurons. Thus p75^{NTR} is expected to interact physically with trk-B and trk-C on the cell surface of motoneurons, and only part if any of the p75^{NTR} transmembrane molecule receptors should exist separately and function independently as cell death receptors on these cells. In the latter case, one would expect that NGF signaling through p75^{NTR} should also reduce the survival response mediated through CNTF or GDNF receptors. However, even high quantities of NGF (20 ng/ml) known to saturate low-affinity receptors on neuronal cells [88] did not reduce CNTF- and GDNF-mediated survival of motoneurons. This was surprising insofar, as the CNTF-mediated survival response of embryonic chick mesencephalic trigeminal neurons was reduced by NGF [20]. We can exclude the possibility that CNTF and GDNF downregulate p75^{NTR} expression in motoneurons, as motoneurons treated either with CNTF, GDNF, or BDNF showed similar intensities of p75^{NTR} immunostaining after 5 days in culture. Thus, we conclude that the role of p75^{NTR} in neuronal cells differs depending on cell type and developmental stage. Whether such differences are caused by the presence or absence of downstream-effectors of trk and p75^{NTR} signaling, or simply by the fact that apoptosis through p75^{NTR} requires higher expression levels than those found in motoneurons from E14 mouse spinal cord, remains to be seen.

Conclusion: implications for therapeutic approaches to improve neuroregeneration after motor nerve lesion

Most clinical trials with neurotrophic factors in neurological disorders like amyotrophic lateral scerosis or diabetic neuropathy have failed so far [2, 3, 12, 54, 67, 100]. Side effects which became detectable in particular after systemic treatment appeared intolerable and/or the clinical improvements were lower than expected [27]. This disappointment has reduced enthusiasm in further clinical tests significantly, and careful retrospective evaluation of possible reasons may help to learn how future trials could be designed for more success. Although this analysis is not yet completed, it becomes clear that the problems have to be sought on several levels. Systemic application leads to side effects, in particular in nonneuronal tissues such as liver where receptor for LIF are expressed, and expression at sites close to the cell bodies could lead to reduced fiber outgrowth to the denervated target tissue by attracting growth cones to the delivery site for but not the initial routes of axonal projection. Thus the mode of application appears highly critical, so that new techniques for delivery have to be developed. Increasing evidence suggests that the distribution of receptors in various compartments of the neuronal cell membrane influences downstream signalling pathways. For example, activation of src and related molecules by receptors for the GDNF family preferentially occurs in lipid-enriched membrane departments. This might have implications on the cellular effects of such factors when applied at sites either close to the cell body or the growth cone of the regenerating axon. Moreover, one neurotrophic factor might not provide all signals which are necessary for survival and neurite regrowth. As discussed above, CNTF and BDNF in combination show supraadditive effects on inhibition of motoneuron atrophy after prolonged periods of peripheral nerve lesion. Other problems which need to be resolved in more detail are differential requirements for signalling pathways in developing and adult neurons. Pathways which are responsible for survival of embryonic motoneurons could take over other functions after birth. Pathways such as activation of Stat-3 which are important for neural differentiation could become increasingly involved in protecting neurons from lesion-induced cell death in the adult.

Another strategy to develop new treatment for lesioned motoneurons is the search for small molecules which stimulate specific cellular pathways which promote survival and axon growth. However, such approaches depend on the definition of specific molecular screening targets. For example, general stimulation of tyrosine kinase signalling is expected to result in uncontrolled growth of many cell types in which tyrosine kinase receptors transduce mitogenic signals. Thus, the search for master regulators in the signalling cascades which promote a survival signal rather than a mitotic signal is of eminent importance. Findings that neurotrophic factors specifically upregulate members of the IAP gene family of caspase-inhibitory molecules or that B-Raf but not C-Raf is required for neuronal survival could provide first ideas on targets for screening of such molecules with specific survival promoting activity. Together with the search for signals which specifically stimulate axon growth, these strategies could ultimately result in better tools to influence regeneration after severe nerve trauma.

Acknowledgments

Work in the author's lab is supported by the Deutsche Forschungsgemeinschaft, Grant To61/8-4, SFB 581, TP B1 and B3 and BMBF 01KO9705.

References

1. Aletta JM (1994) Differential effect of NGF and EGF on ERK in neuronally differentiated PC12 cells. Neuroreport 5: 2090–2092
2. ALS CNTF Treatment Study (ACTS) group (1996) A double-blind placebo-controlled clinical trial of subcutaneous recombinant human ciliary neurotrophic factor (rhCNTF) in amyotrophic lateral sclerosis. Neurology 46: 1244–1249
3. ALS CNTF Treatment Study [ACTS] Group (1995) Phase II–III double blind, placebo-controlled clinical trial of subcutaneous administration od recombinant human ciliary neurotrophic factor (rHCNTF) in Amyotrophic Lateral Sclerosis. Neurology 45 [Suppl] 4: A448
4. Arakawa Y, Sendtner M, Thoenen H (1990) Survival effect of ciliary neurotrophic factor (CNTF) on chick embryonic motoneurons in culture: comparison with other neurotrophic factors and cytokines. J Neurosci 10: 3507–3515
5. Baloh RH, Tansey MG, Golden J, Creedon DJ, Heuckeroth RO, Keck CL, Zimonjic DB, Popescu NC, Johnson EM Jr, Milbrandt J (1997) TrnR2, a novel receptor that mediates neurturin and GDNF signaling through Ret. Neuron 18: 793–802
6. Baloh RH, Tansey MG, Lampe PA, Fahrner TJ, Enomoto H, Simburger KS, Leitner ML, Araki T, Johnson EM Jr, Milbrandt J (1998) Artemin, a novel member of the GDNF ligand family, supports peripheral and central neurons and signals through the GFRalpha3-RET receptor complex. Neuron 21: 1291–1302
7. Bamji SX, Majdan M, Pozniak CD, Belliveau DJ, Aloyz R, Kohn J, Causing CG, Miller FD (1998) The p75 neurotrophin receptor mediates neuronal apoptosis and is essential for naturally occuring sympathetic neuron death. J Cell Biol 140: 911–923
8. Bar-Sagi D, Feramisco JR (1985) Microinjection of the ras oncogene protein into PC12 cells induces morphological differentiation. Cell 42: 841–848
9. Barde YA (1990) The nerve growth factor family. Prog Growth Factor Res 2: 237–248
10. Baxter RM, Cohen P, Obermeier A, Ullrich A, Downes CP, Doza YN (1995) Phosphotyrosine residues in the nerve-growth-factor receptor (Trk-A). Their role in the activation of inositolphospholipid metabolism and protein kinase cascades in phaeochromocytoma (PC12) cells. Eur J Biochem 234: 84–91

11. Borasio GD, Markus A, Wittinghofer A, Barde YA, Heumann R (1993) Involvement of ras p21 in neurotrophin-induced response of sensory, but not sympathetic neurons. J Cell Biol 121: 665–672
12. Bradley WG and The BDNF Study Group (1995) A phase I/II study of recombinant human brain-derived neurotrophic factor in patients with amyotrophic lateral sclerosis. Ann Neurol 38: 971
13. Brunet A, Bonni A, Zigmond MJ, Lin MZ, Juo P, Hu LS, Anderson MJ, Arden KC, Blenis J, Greenberg ME (1999) Akt promotes cell survival by phosphorylating and inhibiting a Forkhead transcription factor. Cell 96: 857–868
14. Cardone MH, Roy N, Stennicke HR, Salvesen GS, Franke TF, Stanbridge E, Frisch S, Reed JC (1998) Regulation of cell death protease caspase-9 by phosphorylation. SCI 282: 1318–1321
15. Carter BD, Zirrgiebel U, Barde YA (1995) Differential regulation of p21ras activation in neurons by nerve growth factor and brain-derived neurotrophic factor. J Biol Chem 270: 21751–21757
16. Cattaneo E, Pelicci PG (1998) Emerging roles for SH2/PTB-containing Shc adaptor proteins in the developing mammalian brain. Trends Neurosci 21: 476–481
17. Chao M, Casaccia-Bonnefil P, Carter B, Chittka A, Kong H, Yoon SO (1998) Neurotrophin receptors: mediators of life and death. Brain Res Brain Res Rev 26: 295–301
18. Conti L, De Fraja C, Gulisano M, Migliaccio E, Govoni S, Cattaneo E (1997) Expression and activation of SH2/PTB-containing ShcA adaptor protein reflects the pattern of neurogenesis in the mammalian brain. Proc Natl Acad Sci USA 94: 8185–8190
19. Datta SR, Dudek H, Tao X, Masters S, Fu H, Gotoh Y, Greenberg ME (1997) Akt phosphorylation of BAD couples survival signals to the cell-intrinsic death machinery. Cell 91: 231–241
20. Davey F, Davies AM (1998) TrkB signalling inhibits p75-mediated apoptosis induced by nerve growth factor in embryonic proprioceptive neurons. Curr Biol 8: 915–918
21. Dechant G, Tsoulfas P, Parada LF, Barde YA (1997) The neurotrophin receptor p75 binds neurotrophin-3 on sympathetic neurons with high affinity and specificity. J Neurosci 17: 5281–5287
22. Deckwerth TL, Easton RM, Knudson CM, Korsmeyer SJ, Johnson EM Jr (1998) Placement of the BCL2 family member BAX in the death pathway of sympathetic neurons activated by trophic factor deprivation. Exp Neurol 152: 150–162
23. Deshmukh M, Johnson EM Jr (1998) Evidence of a novel event during neuronal death: development of competence-to-die in response to cytoplasmic cytochrome c [see comments]. Neuron 21: 695–705
24. Deveraux QL, Roy N, Stennicke HR, Van Arsdale T, Zhou Q, Srinivasula SM, Alnemri ES, Salvesen GS, Reed JC (1998) IAPs block apoptotic events induced by caspase-8 and cytochrome c by direct inhibition of distinct caspases. EMBO J 17: 2215–2223
25. Devereaux QL, Takahashi R, Salvesen GS, Reed JC (1997) X-linked IAP is a direct inhibitor of cell-death proteases. Nature 388: 300–304
26. Digby MR, Kimpton WG, York JJ, Connick TE, Lowenthal JW (1996) ITA, a vertebrate homologue of IAP that is expressed in T lymphocytes. DNA Cell Biol 15: 981–988
27. Dittrich F, Thoenen H, Sendtner M (1994) Ciliary neurotrophic factor: pharmakokinetics and acute phase response. Ann Neurol 35: 151–163
28. Dubois-Dauphin M, Frankowski H, Tsujimoto Y, Huarte J, Martinou JC (1994) Neonatal motoneurons overexpressing the *bcl-2* protooncogene in transgenic mice are protected from axotomy-induced cell death. Proc Natl Acad Sci USA 91: 3309–3313
29. Dudek H, Datta SR, Franke TF, Birnbaum MJ, Yao R, Cooper GM, Segal RA, Kaplan DR, Greenberg ME (1997) Regulation of neuronal survival by the serine-threonine protein kinase Akt. SCI 275: 661–665
30. Ebens A, Brose K, Leonardo ED, Hanson MGJ, Bladt F, Birchmeier C, Barres BA, Tessier-Lavigne M (1996) Hepatocyte growth factor/scatter factor is an axonal chemoattractant and a neurotrophic factor for spinal motor neurons. Neuron 17: 1157–1172
31. Edgar D, Timpl R, Thoenen H (1984) The heparin-binding domain of laminin is responsible for its effects on neurite outgrowth and neuronal survival. EMBO J 3: 1463–1468
32. Elson GC, Lelievre E, Guillet C, Chevalier S, Plun-Favreau H, Froger J, Suard I, de Coignac AB, Delneste Y, Bonnefoy JY, Gauchat JF, Gascan H (2000) CLF associates with CLC to form a functional heteromeric ligand for the CNTF receptor complex. Nat Neurosci 3: 867–872
33. Erhardt P, Troppmair J, Rapp UR, Cooper GM (1995) Differential regulation of Raf-1 and B-Raf and Ras-dependent activation of mitogen-activated protein kinase by cyclic AMP in PC12 cells. Mol Cell Biol 15: 5524–5530
34. Ernfors P, Hallböök F, Ebendal T, Shooter EM, Radeke MJ, Misko TP, Persson H (1988) Developmental and regional expression of β-nerve growth factor receptor mRNA in the chick and rat. Neuron 1: 983–996
35. Ferri CC, Moore FA, Bisby MA (1998) Effects od facial nerve injury on mouse motoneurons lacking the p75 low-affinity neurotrophin receptor. J Neurobiol 34: 1–9
36. Finkbeiner S, Tavazoie SF, Maloratsky A, Jacobs KM, Harris KM, Greenberg ME (1997) CREB: a major mediator of neuronal neurotrophin responses. Neuron 19: 1031–1047
37. Frade JM, Barde YA (1998) Microglia-derived Nerve Growth Factor causes cell death in the developing retina. Neuron 20: 35–42
38. Frade JM, Barde YA (1999) Genetic evidence for cell death mediated by nerve growth factor and the neurotrophin receptor p75 in the developing mouse retina and spinal cord. Development 126: 683–690
39. Frade JM, Rodriguez Tebar A, Barde YA (1996) Induction of cell death by endogenous nerve growth factor through its p75 receptor. Nature 383: 166–168
40. Friedman WJ, Greene LA (1999) Neurotrophin signaling via Trks and p75. Exp Cell Res 253: 131–142
41. Gravel C, Götz R, Lorrain A, Sendtner M (1997) Adenoviral gene transfer of ciliary neurotrophic factor and brain-derived neurotrophic factor leads to longterm survival of axotomized motoneurons. Nature Medicine 3: 765–770
42. Greene LA, Kaplan DR (1995) Early events in neurotrophin signalling via Trk and p75 receptors. Curr Opin Neurobiol 5: 579–587
43. Grewal SS, Horgan AM, York RD, Withers GS, Banker GA, Stork PJ (2000) Neuronal Calcium activates a Rap1 and B-Raf signaling pathway via the cyclic adenosine monophosphate-dependent protein kinase. J Biol Chem 275: 3722–3728
44. Grieshammer U, Lewandoski M, Prevette D, Oppenheim RW, Martin GR, Pettmann B, Henderson CE (1998) Muscle-specific cell ablation conditional upon Cre-mediated DNA recombination in transgenic mice leads to massive spinal and cranial motoneuron loss Neuronal cell death. Neuron 20: 633–647
45. Hamburger V (1934) The effects of wing bud extirpation on the development of the central nervous system in chick embryos. J Exp Zool 68: 449–494

46. Hamburger V (1958) Regression versus peripheral control of differentiation in motor hyperplasia. Am J Anat 102: 365–410
47. Henderson CE, Camu W, Mettling C, Gouin A, Poulsen K, Karihaloo M, Rullamas J, Evans T, McMahon SB, Armanini MP, Berkemeier L, Phillips HS, Rosenthal A (1993) Neurotrophins promote motor neuron survival and are present in embryonic limb bud. Nature 363: 266–270
48. Henderson CE, Phillips HS, Pollock RA, Davies AM, Lemeulle C, Armanini M, Simpson LC, Moffet B, Vandlen RA, Koliatsos VE *et al* (1994) GDNF: a potent survival factor for motoneurons present in peripheral nerve and muscle. SCI 266: 1062–1064
49. Hughes RA, Sendtner M, Thoenen H (1993) Members of several gene families influence survival of rat motoneurons in vitro and in vivo. J Neurosci Res 36(6): 663–671
50. Jablonka S, Schrank B, Kralewski M, Rossoll W, Sendtner M (2000) Reduced survival motor neuron (Smn) gene dose in mice leads to motor neuron degeneration: an animal model for spinal muscular atrophy type III [in process citation]. Hum Mol Genet 9: 341–346
51. Kalb RG, Lidow MS, Halsted M, Hockfield S (1992) N-Methyl-D-aspartate receptors are transiently expressed in the developing spinal cord ventral horn. Proc Natl Acad Sci USA 89: 8502–8506
52. Klein RD, Sherman D, Ho WH, Stone D, Bennett GL, Moffat B, Vandlen R, Simmons L, Gu Q, Hongo JA, Devaux B, Poulson K, Armanini M, Nozaki C, Asai N, Goddard A, Phllips H, Henderson CE, Takahashi M, Rosenthal A (1997) A GPI-linked protein that interacts with Ret to form a candidate neurturin receptor. Nature 387: 717–721
53. Knudson CM, Tung KS, Tourtellotte WG, Brown GA, Korsmeyer SJ (1995) Bax-deficient mice with lymphoid hyperplasia and male germ cell death. SCI 270: 96–99
54. Lai EC, Felice BW, Festoff BW *et al* (1995) A double-blind, placebo-controlled study of recombinant human insulin-like growth factor in the treatment of amyotrophic lateral sclerosis. Ann Neurol 38: 971
55. Levi-Montalcini R (1950) The origin and development of the visceral system in the spinal cord of the chick embryo. J Morphol 253–284
56. Mahadeo D, Kaplan L, Chao MV, Hempstead BL (1994) High affinity nerve growth factor binding displays a faster rate of association than $p140^{trk}$ binding. Implications for multi-subunit polypeptide receptors. J Biol Chem 269: 6884–6891
57. Majdan M, Lachance C, Gloster A, Aloyz R, Zeindler C, Bamji S, Bhakar A, Belliveau D, Fawcett J, Miller FD, Barker PA (1997) Transgenic mice expressing the intracellular domain of the p75 neurotrophin receptor undergo neuronal apoptosis. J Neurosci 17: 6988–6998
58. Martinou JC, Dubois-Dauphin M, Staple JK, Rodriguez I, Frankowski H, Missotten M, Albertini P, Talabot D, Catsicas S, Pietra C, Huarte J (1994) Overexpression of BCL-2 in transgenic mice protects neurons from naturally occurring cell death and experimental ischemia. Neuron 13: 1017–1030
59. Meakin SO, Shooter EM (1992) The nerve growth factor family of receptors. TINS 15: 323–331
60. Metzger F, Kulik A, Sendtner M, Ballanyi K (2000) Contribution of Ca(2+)-permeable AMPA/KA receptors to glutamate-induced Ca(2+) rise in embryonic lumbar motoneurons in situ. J Neurophysiol 83: 50–59
61. Metzger F, Wiese S, Sendtner M (1998) Effect of glutamate on dendritic growth in embryonic rat motoneurons. J Neurosci 18: 1735–1742
62. Metzstein MM, Hengartner MO, Tsung N, Ellis RE, Horvitz HR (1996) Transcriptional regulator of programmed cell death encoded by Caenorhabditis elegans gene ces-2. Nature 382: 545–547
63. Meyer-Franke A, Wilkinson GA, Kruttgen A, Hu M, Munro E, Hanson MG Jr, Reichardt LF, Barres BA (1998) Depolarization and cAMP elevation rapidly recruit TrkB to the plasma membrane of CNS neurons. Neuron 21: 681–693
64. Meyer Franke A, Kaplan MR, Pfrieger FW, Barres BA (1995) Characterization of the signaling interactions that promote the survival and growth of developing retinal ganglion cells in culture. Neuron 15: 805–819
65. Michaelidis TM, Sendtner M, Cooper JD, Airaksinen M, Holtmann B, Meyer M, Thoenen H (1996) Inactivation of the bcl-2 gene results in progressive degeneration of motoneurons, sensory and sypathetic neurons during early postnatal development. Neuron 17: 75–89
66. Milbrandt J, de Sauvage FJ, Fahrner TJ, Baloh RH, Leitner ML, Tansey MG, Lampe PA, Heuckeroth RO, Kotzbauer PT, Simburger KS, Golden JP, Davies JA, Vejsada R, Kato AC, Hynes M, Sherman D, Nishimura M, Wang LC, Vandlen R, Moffat B, Klein RD, Poulsen K, Gray C, Garces A, Johnson EMJ, *et al*, Johnson EM Jr (1998) Persephin, a novel neurotrophic factor related to GDNF and neurturin. Neuron 20: 245–253
67. Miller RG, Armon C, Bahron R, Bryan W, Goodpasture J, Parry G, Petajan J, Ross M, Stromatt S, ALS SSNJV Study Group (1995) A controlled trial of Recombinant Human Ciliary Neurotrophic Factor (rhCNTF) in Amyotrophic Lateral Sclerosis (ALS). Neurology 45 [Suppl] 4: A280–281
68. Minichiello L, Casagranda F, Tatche RS, Stucky CL, Postigo A, Lewin GR, Davies AM, Klein R (1998) Point mutation in trkB causes loss of NT4-dependent neurons without major effects on diverse BDNF responses. Neuron 21: 335–345
69. Miyata Y, Kashihara Y, Homma S, Kuno M (1986) Effects of nerve growth factor on the survival and synaptic function of Ia sensory neurons axotomized in neonatal rats. J Neurosci 6: 2012–2018
70. Monani UR, Sendtner M, Coovert DD, Parsons DW, Andreassi C, Le TT, Jablonka S, Schrank B, Rossol W, Prior TW, Morris GE, Burghes AH (2000) The human centromeric survival motor neuron gene (SMN2) rescues embryonic lethality in Smn(−/−) mice and results in a mouse with spinal muscular atrophy. Hum Mol Genet 9: 333–339
71. Nagata S (1997) Apoptosis by death factor. *Cell* 88: 355–365
72. Nakamura T, Sanokawa R, Sasaki Y, Ayusawa D, Oishi M, Mori N (1996) N-Shc: a neural-specific adapter molecule that mediates signaling from neurotrophin/Trk to Ras/Mapk pathway. Oncogene 1111–1121
73. Nakashima K, Taga T (1998) gp130 and the IL-6 family of cytokines: signaling mechanisms and thrombopoietic activities. Semin Hematol 35: 210–221
74. Neff NT, Prevette D, Houenou LJ, Lewis ME, Glicksman MA, Yin QW, Oppenheim RW (1993) Insulin-like growth factors: Putative muscle-derived trophic agents that promote motoneuron survival. J Neurobiol 24: 1578–1588
75. Newmeyer DD, Green DR (1998) Surviving the cytochrome seas. Neuron 21: 653–655
76. Novak KD, Prevette D, Wang S, Gould TW, Oppenheim RW (2000) Hepatocyte growth factor/scatter factor is a neurotrophic survival factor for lumbar but not for other somatic motoneurons in the chick embryo. J Neurosci 20: 326–337
77. O'Connor TM, Wyttenbach CR (1974) Cell death of the embryonic chick spinal cord. J Cell Biol 60: 448–459
78. Obermeier A, Bradshaw RA, Seedorf K, Choidas A, Schlessinger J, Ullrich A (1994) Neuronal differentiation signals are

controlled by nerve growth factor receptor/Trk binding sites for SHC and PLCgamma. EMBO J 13: 1585–1590
79. Obermeier A, Lammers R, Wiesmuller KH, Jung G, Schlessinger J, Ullrich A (1993) Identification of Trk binding sites for SHC and phosphatidylinositol 3′-kinase and formation of a multimeric signaling complex. J Biol Chem 268: 22963–22966
80. Okado N, Oppenheim RW (1984) Cell death of motoneurons in the chick embryo spinal cord IX, the loss of motoneurons following removal of afferent inputs. J Neurosci 4: 1639–1652
81. Oppenheim RW (1985) Naturally occurring cell death during neural development. Trends in Neuroscience 8: 487–493
82. Oppenheim RW, Cole T, Prevette D (1989) Early regional variations in motoneuron numbers arise by differential proliferation in the chick embryo spinal cord. Dev Biol 133: 468–474
83. Ozes ON, Mayo LD, Gustin JA, Pfeffer SR, Pfeffer LM, Donner DB (1999) NF-kappaB activation by tumour necrosis factor requires the Akt serine-threonine kinase. Nature 401: 82–85
84. Pennica D, Shaw KJ, Swanson TA, Moore MW, Shelton DL, Zioncheck KA, Rosenthal A, Taga T, Paoni NF, Wood WI (1995) Cardiotrophin-1. Biological activities and binding to the leukemia inhibitory factor receptor/gp130 signaling complex. J Biol Chem 270: 10915–10922
85. Qin-Wei Y, Johnson J, Prevette D, Oppenheim RW (1994) Cell death of spinal motoneurons in the chick embryo following deafferentiation: Rescue effects of tissue extracts, soluble proteins, and neurotrophic agents. J Neurosci 14: 7629–7640
86. Raoul C, Henderson CE, Pettmann B (1999) Programmed cell death of embryonic motoneurons triggered through the Fas death receptor. J Cell Biol 147: 1049–1062
87. Riethmacher D, Sonnenberg-Riethmacher E, Brinkmann V, Vamaai T, Lewin GR, Birchmeier C (1997) Severe neuropathies in mice with targeted mutations in the ErbB3 receptor. Nature 725–730
88. Rodriguez-Tébar A, Dechant G, Barde YA (1990) Binding of brain-derived neurotrophic factor to the nerve growth factor receptor. Neuron 4: 487–492
89. Romashkova JA, Makarov SS (1999) NF-kappaB is a target of AKT in anti-apoptotic PDGF signalling. Nature 401: 86–90
90. Rothstein JD (1995) Excitotoxic mechanisms in the pathogenesis of amyotrophic lateral sclerosis. Adv Neurol 68: 7–20
91. Roy N, Deveraux QL, Takahashi R, Salvesen GS, Reed JC (1997) The c-IAP-1 and c-IAP-2 proteins are direct inhibitors of specific caspases. EMBO J 16: 6914–6925
92. Segal RA, Greenberg ME (1996) Intracellular signaling pathways activated by neurotrophic factors. Annu Rev Neurosci 19: 463–489
93. Senaldi G, Varnum BC, Sarmiento U, Starnes C, Lile J, Scully S, Guo J, Elliott G, McNinch J, Shaklee CL, Freeman D, Manu F, Simonet WS, Boone T, Chang MS (1999) Novel neurotrophin-1/B cell-stimulating factor-3: A cytokine of the IL-6 family. Proc Natl Acad Sci USA 96: 11458–11463
94. Sendtner M (1998) Neurotrophic factors: effects in modulating properties of the neuromuscular endplate. Cytokine Growth Factor Rev 9: 1–7
95. Sendtner M, Arakawa Y, Stöckli KA, Kreutzberg GW, Thoenen H (1991) Effect of ciliary neurotrophic factor (CNTF) on motoneuron survival. J Cell Sci [Suppl] 15: 103–109
96. Sendtner M, Holtmann B, Kolbeck R, Thoenen H, Barde YA (1992) Brain-derived neurotrophic factor prevents the death of motoneurons in newborn rats after nerve section. Nature 360: 757–758
97. Shi Y, Wang W, Yourey PA, Gohari S, Zukauskas D, Zhang J, Ruben S, Alderson RF (1999) Computational EST database analysis identifies a novel member of the neuropoietic cytokine family. Biochem Biophys Res Commun 262: 132–138
98. Slee EA, Harte MT, Kluck RM, Wolf BB, Casiano CA, Newmeyer DD, Wang HG, Reed JC, Nicholson DW, Alnemri ES, Green DR, Martin SJ (1999) Ordering the Cytochrome c-initiated Caspase Cascade: Hierarchical Activation of Caspases-2, -3, -6, -7, -8, and -10 in a Caspase-9-dependent Manner. J Cell Biol 144: 281–292
99. Stennicke HR, Deveraux QL, Humke EW, Reed JC, Dixit VM, Salvesen GS (1999) Caspase-9 can Be activated without proteolytic processing [in process citation]. J Biol Chem 274: 8359–8362
100. The BDNF Study Group and Bradley W *et al* (1995) Subcutaneous administration of recombinant Brain-derived neurotrophic factor (r-metHuBDNF) in patients with amyotrophic lateral sclerosis. 6th International Symposium on ALS/MND. Dublin, abstract book
101. Tinhofer I, Maly K, Dietl P, Hochholdinger F, Mayr S, Obermeier A, Grunicke HH (1996) Differential Ca2+ signaling induced by activation of the epidermal growth factor and nerve growth factor receptors. J Biol Chem 271: 30505–30509
102. Traverse S, Gomez N, Paterson H, Marshall C, Cohen P (1992) Sustained activation of the mitogen-activated protein (MAP) kinase cascade may be required for differentiation of PC12 cells. Comparison of the effects of nerve growth factor and epidermal growth factor. Biochem J 288 (Pt 2): 351–355
103. Van der Zee CE, Ross GM, Riopelle RJ, Hagg T (1996) Survival of cholinergic forebrain neurons in developing p75NGFR-deficient mice [see comments] [retracted by Hagg T. In: Science 1999 Jul 16; 285(5426): 340]. SCI 274: 1729–1732
104. Vejsada R, Sagot Y, Kato AC (1995) Quantitative comparison of the transient rescue effects of neurotrophic factors on axotomized motoneurons in vivo. Eur J Neurosci 7: 108–115
105. Wakade AR, Edgar D, Thoenen H (1983) Both nerve growth factor and high K concentration support the survival of chick embryo sympathetic neurons. Exp Cell Res 144: 377–384
106. Wang HG, Miyashita T, Takayama S, Sato T, Torigoe T, Krajewski S, Tanaka S, Hovey L, III, Troppmair J, Rapp UR, Reed JC (1994) Apoptosis regulation by interaction of Bcl-2 protein and Raf-1 kinase. Oncogene 9: 2751–2756
107. Wang HG, Rapp UR, Reed JC (1996) Bcl-2 targets the protein kinase Raf-1 to mitochondria. Cell 87: 629–638
108. Wiese S, Digby MR, Gunnersen JM, Götz R, Pei G, Holtmann B, Lowenthal J, Sendtner M (1999) The anti-apoptotic protein ITA is essential for NGF-mediated survival of embryonic chick neurons. Nat Neurosci 2: 978–983
109. Wiese S, Metzger F, Holtmann B, Sendtner M (1999) The role of p75NTR in modulating neurotrophin survival effects in developing motoneurons. Eur J Neurosci 11: 1668–1676
110. Wiese S, Pei G, Karch C, Troppmair J, Holtmann B, Rapp UR, Sendtner M (2001) Specific function of B-Raf in mediating survival of embryonic motoneurons and sensory neurons. Nat Neurosci 4: 137–142
111. Wixler V, Smola U, Schuler M, Rapp U (1996) Differential regulation of Raf isozymes by growth versus differentiation inducing factors in PC12 pheochromocytoma cells. FEBS Lett 385: 131–137
112. Wolf DE, McKinnon CA, Daou MC, Stephens RM, Kaplan DR, Ross AH (1995) Interaction with TrkA immobilizes gp75 in the high affinity nerve growth factor receptor complex. J Biol Chem 270: 2133–2138
113. Yaginuma H, Tomita M, Takashita N, McKay SE, Cardwell C, Yin QW, Oppenheim RW (1996) A novel type of programmed neuronal death in the cervical spinal cord of the chick embryo. J Neurosci 16: 3685–3703
114. Yamamoto Y, Livet J, Polock R, Garces A, Arce V, deLapeyiére O, Henderson C (1997) Hepatocyte groeth factor

(HGF/SF) is a muscle-derived survival factor for a subpopulation of embryonic motoneurons. Development [Suppl] 124: 2903–2913

115. Yeo TT, Chua-Couzens J, Butcher LL, Bredesen DE, Cooper JD, Valletta JS, Mobley WC, Longo FM (1997) Absence of p75NTR causes increased basal forebrain cholinergic neuron size, choline acetyltrasnferase activity, and target innervation. J Neurosci 17: 7594–7605
116. Yeo TT, Chua-Couzens J, Butcher LL, Bredesen DE, Cooper JD, Valletta JS, Mobley WC, Longo FM (1997) Absence of p75NTR causes increased basal forebrain cholinergic neuron size, choline acetyltrasnferase activity, and target innervation. J Neurosci 17: 7594–7605
117. York RD, Yao H, Dillon T, Ellig CL, Eckert SP, McCleskey EW, Stork PJ (1998) Rap1 mediates sustained MAP kinase activation induced by nerve growth factor. Nature 392: 622–626
118. Zurn AD, Baetge EE, Hammang JP, Tan SA, Aebischer P (1994) Glial cell line-derived neurotrophic factor (GDNF), a new neurotrophic factor for motoneurones. Neuroreport 6: 113–118

Correspondence: Michael Sendtner, Institute for Clinical Neurobiology, Josef-Schneider-Str.11, 97080 Würzburg, Germany. e-mail: sendtner@mail.uni-wuerzburg.de

Acta Neurochir (2004) [Suppl] 89: 37–45

Printed in Austria

Genetically modified animals in molecular stroke research

K.-A. Hossmann

Max-Planck-Institute for Neurological Research, Department of Experimental Neurology, Cologne, Germany

Introduction

Brain damage induced by focal interruption of blood flow can be differentiated in two pathophysiologically different categories: a hemodynamic type of injury, resulting in primary necrotic brain damage, and a molecular type of injury which leads to delayed or secondary brain injury [15]. Primary necrotic brain injury occurs when blood flow declines – and remains – below the threshold of energy failure. In anaesthetized laboratory animals, this threshold gradually increases from about 15% of control shortly after the onset of ischemia to about 30% after several hours of vascular occlusion [35].

Delayed or secondary brain damage occurs in regions called "at risk" which are not intact but which have not yet suffered tissue necrosis. In permanent focal ischemia this type of injury evolves in the periinfarct penumbra which, by definition, is the peripheral part of the ischemic territory in which functional activity but not energy metabolism are suppressed [31]. After transient focal ischemia, the area "at risk" is the part of the ischemic territory in which energy metabolism has failed during ischemia but recovers after reversal of the vascular occlusion [32]. With increasing duration of ischemia this region shifts from the central to the peripheral parts of the ischemic territory until – under conditions of irreversible energy failure – it becomes congruent with the penumbra of permanent vascular occlusion [32].

A biochemical hallmark of tissue "at risk" for delayed ischemic injury is the dissociation between maintained (or restored) energy metabolism and suppressed protein synthesis [35]. Another predictor of delayed cell death is the upregulation of *hsp70* mRNA which has been interpreted as evidence for the cytosolic stress response [68]. However, this response is only a marker and not a mediator of injury because translation of HSP70 protein, as induced by sublethal pre-ischemic conditioning, conveys neuroprotection to a subsequent more severe ischemic impact.

Obviously, precise understanding of the mechanisms of delayed ischemic brain injury is of considerable interest for the identification of molecular targets for therapeutic interventions. In the past, research into this field has been mainly accomplished by pharmacological approaches but the difficulties encountered in translating the experimental observations into clinically successful treatment protocols have raised concerns about the relevance of these interventions [25]. More recently, the availability of genetically modified laboratory animals has provided the opportunity to dissect molecular injury pathways in a much more specific way [6]. A rapidly increasing number of laboratories have embarked on this new methodology, and important data have been generated which have helped to clarify complex molecular interactions. However, some of these data are controversial, and the expected identification of a unique injury pathway has not yet succeeded.

Methodological considerations

Gene manipulations are most frequently carried out in mice, either by microinjection of DNA into pronuclei of fertilized oocytes [23] or by introducing foreign genes into embryonic stem cells [74]. The stem cells are microinjected into blastocytes to produce chimeras which are mated with wild-type animals to generate heterozygous – and after further crossbreading – homozygous offsprings. The strains most commonly used are SV129 for the preparation of stem cells and

C57Black for blastocyte injection. However, these strains differ substantially in their susceptibility to cerebral ischemia. In C57Black mice ligation of the middle cerebral artery (MCA) results in brain infarcts which are at least 30% larger than in the SV129 strain [12; 52]. Angioarchitectural studies from our laboratory reveiled that this difference is due to the larger vascular territory supplied by the MCA [51] (Fig. 1). On the other hand, C57Black mice are less susceptible to excitotoxic injury [65] and exhibit more robust vasoreactivity [21] which may partly counteract the angioarchitectural disadvantage of this strain.

Obviously, strain differences may interfere with the effects of targeted mutations as long as the genetic background of the transgenic animals has not become homologous. However, as full homology requires backcrossings for 12 generations which takes about two years, only few of the published studies fulfill this requirement.

Another methodological problem for the comparison of ischemic injury in transgenic and wild type animals is the possibility of differences in body weight. Ischemic infarcts are most widely produced by intraluminal thread insertion into the MCA but to achieve consistent occlusion the tip diameter of the filament has to be adjusted to the vessel size which, in turn, varies as a function of body weight [33] (Fig. 2). Using the same filament for MCA occlusion in differently sized animals may, therefore, produce different severities of ischemia and, in consequence, differences in stroke outcome.

Finally, the choice of the experimental stroke model may have profound influences on the effect on gene manipulation. In particular, transient and permanent focal ischemia trigger different molecular injury pathways [31; 32], and even within the same category of ischemia, the contribution of primary and secondary injury mechanisms varies, depending on the severity and duration of ischemia and/or reperfusion (Figs. 3, 4). Deletion or overexpression of the same gene,

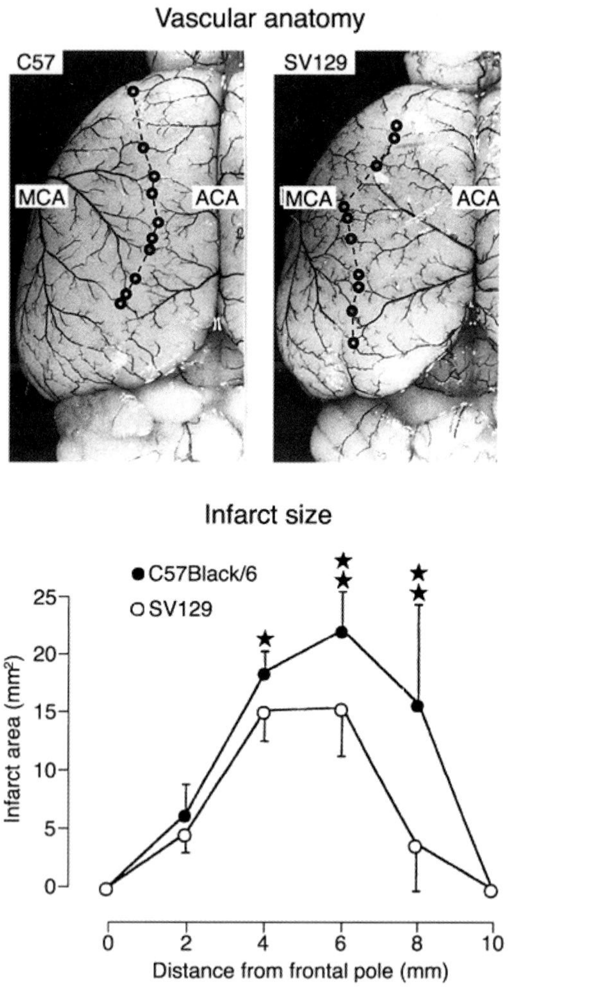

Fig. 1. Difference in mouse strain susceptibility to stroke. Above: Latex infusion of cerebral vasculature of C57Black (left) and SV129 (right) animals. The line of anastomoses between the supplying territories of the anterior cerebral artery *(ACA)* and middle cerebral artery *(MCA)* is marked by the dotted line. The peripheral shift of the line of anastomoses in C57Black mice reflects the larger MCA territory in this strain. Below: Comparison of infarct size in C57Black and SV129 mice. Infarct areas were measured by planimetry on coronal slices at the indicated planes. Mean infarct volumes as calculated by integration was significantly larger in the C57 Black strain (modified from Maeda *et al* [51, 52])

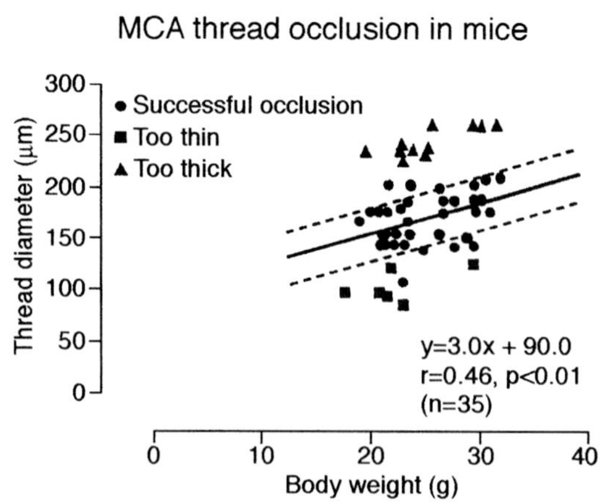

Fig. 2. Relationship between body weight and thread size for successful occlusion of the middle cerebral artery in mice. The narrow range of successful occlusion demonstrates that filament size has to be precisely matched to body weight for obtaining reproducible infarcts (modified from Hata *et al* 1998 [33])

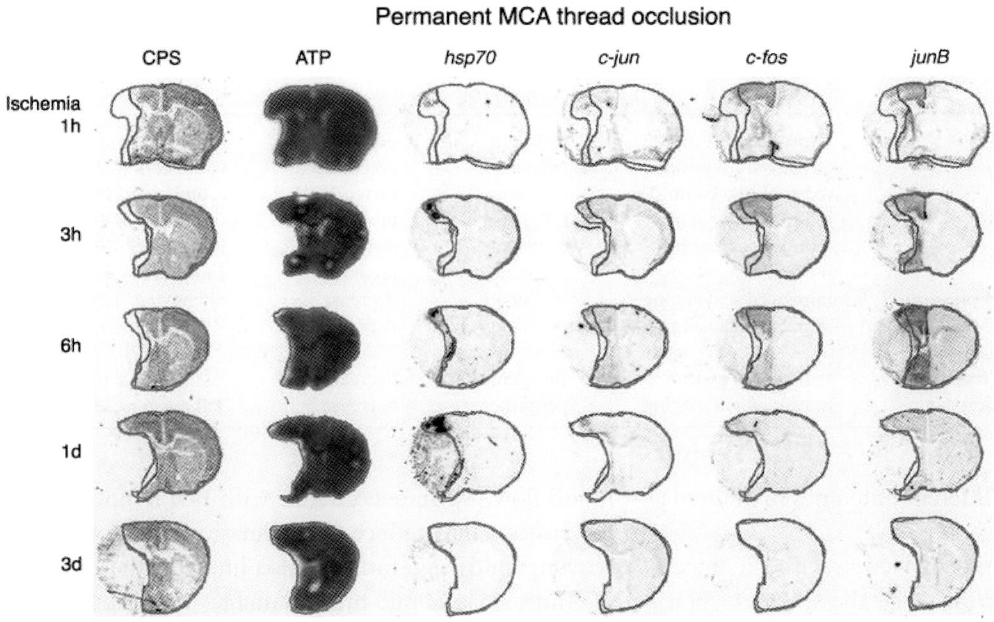

Fig. 3. Dynamics of brain infarct evolution in C57Black mice during permanent middle cerebral artery *(MCA)* occlusion. Multiparametric imaging of cerebral protein synthesis *(CPS)*, ATP content and the expression of *hsp70*, *c-jun*, *c-fos*, and *junB* mRNA in representative brain sections at the level of the caudate-putamen. The outlines of preserved ATP and CPS have been superimposed to demarcate the core from the penumbra of the evolving infarct. Note gradual expansion of infarct core (defined as ATP-depleted tissue) into the penumbra (defined as tissue with suppressed CPS but preserved ATP), and differential expression of *hsp70* and immediate early genes in the penumbra and the peri-infarct normal brain tissue (modified from Hata *et al* 2000a [31])

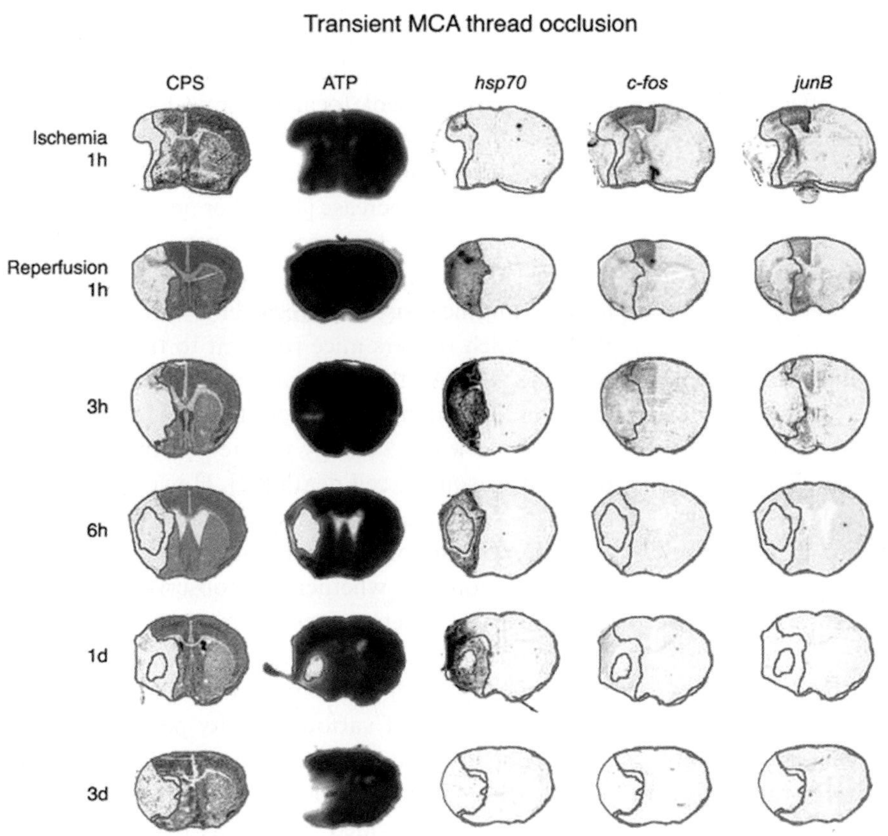

Fig. 4. Evolution of brain injury in C57Black mice after transient focal ischemia. Multiparametric images of cerebral protein synthesis *(CPS)*, tissue ATP content and of *hsp70*, *c-fos*, and *junB* mRNAs in representative brain sections at the level of the caudate-putamen after middle cerebral artery occlusion for one hour. The outlines of preserved ATP and CPS have been superimposed to demarcate the metabolically impaired areas from the normal brain tissue (modified from Hata *et al* 2000b [32])

Table 1. *Gene manipulations interfering with free radical induced injury*

Gene manipulation	Expected effect on free radicals	MCA occlusion	Effect on infarct size	Reference
Cu/Zn-SOD overexpression	improved scavenging	transient	decrease	Kinouchi *et al* 1991 [41]
Cu/Zn-SOD overexpression	improved scavenging	permanent	no change	Chan *et al* 1993 [9]
Cu/Zn-SOD deletion	reduced scavenging	transient	increase	Kondo *et al* 1997 [43]
Cu/ZN-SOD inactivation	reduced scavenging	transient	increase	Guo *et al* 2000 [26]
Mn-SOD deletion	reduced scavenging	transient	decrease	Keller *et al* 1998 [40]
Mn-SOD inactivation	reduced scavenging	permanent	increase	Fujimura *et al* 1999 [22]
APO (apolipoprotein) E3 overexpression	improved scavenging	transient	decrease	Sheng *et al* 1999 [69]
GP (glutathione peroxidase) overexpression	improved scavenging	transient	decrease	Weisbrot-Lefkowitz *et al* 1997 [77]
X-GCD (dysfunctional NADP oxidase)	reduced formation	transient	decrease	Walder *et al* 1997 [75]
TRX (thioreduxin) overexpression	improved scavenging	permanent	decrease	Takagi *et al* 1999 [73]

may, therefore, result in different outcomes in different models.

From a conceptual point of view, such differences are of considerable importance for the search of new molecular targets for stroke therapy. Under clinical conditions, blood flow disturbances associated with stroke are heterogenous, covering all possible combinations from minor to severe flow reduction, followed by different rates of reperfusion after greatly varying delays. As the precise profile of flow changes cannot be easily assessed in each patient, only those molecular targets will be of interest for clinical treatment which relate to an universal model-independent mechanism of ischemic cell death. Comparing the effect of transgenic mutation in different experimental models may, therefore, help to identify such targets.

Modulation of stroke impact in genetically modified animals

A summary of published data on the effect of gene manipulations on brain infarct size is given in the tables (please note that multiple publications from the same laboratory are cited only once). To facilitate comparisons between the various studies, targeted injury mechanisms were classified into various categories which, however, reflect more the current research interests than a systematic categorization of injury pathways.

One of the earliest topics addressed by using genetically modified animals was free radical-induced brain damage (Table 1). Free radicals are generated mainly during reoxygenation after temporary oxygen deprivation and, therefore, are of particular pathophysiological significance following transient interruption of blood flow [8]. In accordance with this hypothesis interventions that reduce the formation or improve the scavenging of free radicals also improve the outcome of transient ischemic brain damage. In permanent ischemia, free radical induced injury is probably restricted to areas in which residual blood flow oscillates around the threshold of metabolic disturbance. This explains that during permanent ischemia manipulation of the radical scavenging capacity either does [22; 73] or does not [9] result in the expected modulation of brain damage.

Apoptosis, in contrast to free radicals, is thought to contribute to the evolution of injury after both permanent and transient focal ischemia [54], but some of the reported data are controversial (Table 2). For instance, overexpression of the anti-apoptotic gene bcl-2 led to either decrease [44; 53] or no change [3; 78], and deletion of the anti-apoptotic gene p53 either decreased [13] or increased [50] ischemic damage. There is also an inconsistency regarding the deletion of PARP which renders mice resistant to transient focal ischemia [17]. As this nuclear enzyme uses NAD for repair of DNA damage, the resulting NAD depletion – which could lead to energy failure – is thought to be the final reason for cell death [61]. However, simultaneous measurements of the tissue content of NAD and ATP do not support this contention [60]. It is, therefore, questionable whether the observed beneficial effect of PARP deletion uses this mechanism for tissue protection.

Genetically modified animals have also been used for the dissection of various toxicity pathways which have been implicated to mediate ischemic or post-ischemic brain damage (Table 3). In particular, evidence has been provided in support of molecular injury mediated by nitric oxide (NO), glutamate, tissue

Table 2. *Apoptosis-associated gene manipulations*

Gene-manipulation	Expected effect on apoptosis	MCA occlusion	Effect on infarct size	Reference
bcl-2 deletion	facilitation	transient	increase	Hata *et al* 1999 [30]
bcl-2 overexpression	inhibition	transient	decrease	Lawrence *et al* 1996 [44]
bcl-2 overexpression	inhibition	permanent	no change	Bilbao *et al* 2000 [3]
bcl-2 overexpression	inhibition	permanent	no change	Wiessner *et al* 1999 [78]
bcl-2 overexpression	inhibition	permanent	decrease	Martinou *et al* 1994 [53]
bcl-X_L overexpression	inhibition	permanent	decrease	Wiessner *et al* 1999 [78]
p53 deletion	inhibition	permanent	decrease	Crumrine *et al* 1994 [13]
p53 deletion	inhibition	transient	increase	Maeda *et al* 2001 [50]
ICE deletion	inhibition	permanent	decrease	Schielke *et al* 1998 [66]
ICE deletion	inhibition	permanent	decrease	Yang *et al* 1999 [79]
ICE negative inhibitor	inhibition	permanent	decrease	Friedlander *et al* 1997 [20]
ICE negative inhibitor	inhibition	transient	decrease	Hara *et al* 1997 [27]
lpr (fas loss of function) mutation	inhibition	transient	decrease	Rosenbaum *et al* 2000 [63]
p50 (NF-kappaB subunit) deletion	inhibition	transient	decrease	Schneider *et al* 1999 [67]
PARP deletion	inhibition	transient	decrease	Eliasson *et al* 1997 [17]
E2F1 (transcription factor) deletion	inhibition	transient	decrease	MacManus *et al* 1999 [48]

Table 3. *Gene manipulations interfering with neurotoxicity*

Gene manipulation	Effect on neurotoxicity	MCA occlusion	Effect on infarct size	Reference
NR2C (NMDA receptor) deletion	reduced excitotoxicity	permanent	decrease	Kadotani *et al* 1998 [39]
NR2A (NMDA receptor) deletion	reduced excitotoxicity	transient	decrease	Morikawa *et al* 1998 [56]
AMPA-receptor overexpression	increased excitotoxicity	permanent	increase	Le *et al* 1997 [45]
nNOS deletion	reduced NO toxicity	permanent	decrease	Huang *et al* 1994 [37]
nNOS deletion	reduced NO toxicity	transient	decrease	Ferriero *et al* 1996 [19]
nNOS deletion	reduced NO toxicity	transient	decrease	Hara *et al* 1996 [28]
iNOS deletion	reduced NO toxicity	permanent	decrease	Nagayama *et al* 1999 [58]
iNOS deletion	reduced NO toxicity	permanent	decrease	Iadecola *et al* 1997 [38]
iNOS deletion	reduced NO toxicity	permanent	decrease	Zhao *et al* 2000 [81]
eNOS deletion	reduced NO toxicity but impaired blood flow	permanent	increase	Huang *et al* 1996 [36]
t-PA deletion	reduced excitotoxicity	transient	decrease	Wang *et al* 1998 [76]
t-PA deletion	reduced excitotoxicity	permanent	decrease	Nagai *et al* 1999 [57]
t-PA deletion	reduced excitotoxicity but impaired recirculation	transient	increase	Tabrizi *et al* 1999 [72]
uPA deletion	reduced excitotoxicity	permanent	no change	Nagai *et al* 1999 [57]
PAI (plasminogen activator inhibitor)-1 deletion	increased excitotoxicity	permanent	increase	Nagai *et al* 1999 [57]
MT (metallothionin)-1 overexpression	reduced Zinc toxicity	transient	decrease	Campagne *et al* 1999 [7]

plasminogen activator (t-PA) or zinc. The genetic approach was particularly successful in elucidating the dual role of NO, depending on the cellular origin of generation [14]. At the vascular level NO is protective because stimulation of endothelial NOS produces vasodilation and, as a consequence, improves collateral blood supply [46]. Stimulation of neuronal or inducible NOS, in contrast, promotes ischemic injury because parenchymal increase of NO facilitates the formation of peroxynitrite [16]. Similarly, t-PA may exert a dual effect by promoting thrombolytic reperfusion but facilitating excitotoxicity [72].

Finally, experiments have been carried out with genetically modified animals to understand the role of various biologically active proteins in modulating ischemia-associated inflammation (Table 4), signalling and stress pathways (Table 5), or other disease-related tissue injury cascades (Table 6). These studies are in general support of established hypotheses on molecular injury pathways but some negative results have been interpreted as evidence to the contrary [11; 29; 47; 50; 64]. However, the methodological constraints cited above may also lead to false negative conclusions, and care should be taken not to overinterpret such data.

Table 4. *Gene manipulations interfering with inflammation*

Gene manipulation	Effect on inflammation	MCA occlusion	Effect on infarct size	Reference
ICAM-1 deletion	reduced neutrophil adhesion	permanent, transient	decrease	Kitagawa *et al* 1998 [42]
ICAM-1 deletion	reduced neutrophil adhesion	transient	decrease	Soriano *et al* 1996 [71]
MCAC-1 deletion	reduced neutrophil adhesion	transient	decrease	Soriano *et al* 1999 [70]
IL-6 deletion	reduced leukocyte activation	transient	no change	Clark *et al* 2000 [11]
IL-10 deletion	reduced immunoresponse	permanent	increase	Grilli *et al* 2000 [24]
TNFR deletion	reduced TNF response	transient	increase	Bruce *et al* 1996 [5]
MMP (matrix-metalloproteinase)-9 deletion	prevention of matrix protein degradation	permanent	decrease	Asahi *et al* 2000 [2]

Table 5. *Gene manipulations interfering with signalling pathways and the cellular stress response*

Gene manipulation	Effect on cellular dysfunction	MCA occlusion	Effect on infarct size	Reference
CREB deletion	reduced cAMP signalling	permanent	no change	Hata *et al* 1998 [29]
SHP2 inactivation	reduced cytokine and growth factor signalling	transient	decrease	Aoki *et al* 2000 [1]
ER alpha deletion	reduced estrogen signalling	transient	no change	Sampai *et al* 2000 [64]
Adenosin (A)2a deletion	reduced adenosine signalling	transient	decrease	Chen *et al* 1999 [10]
MAO–B deletion	reduced monoamine signalling	permanent	no change	Holschneider *et al* 1999 [34]
ODC overexpression	increased polyamine response	transient	no change	Lukkarinen *et al* 1999 [47]
Hsp-70 overexpression	increased stress response	permanent	decrease	Rajdev *et al* 2000 [62]
HO-1 overexpression	improved stress adaptation	permanent	decrease	Panahian *et al* 1999 [59]

Table 6. *Genes interfering with miscellaneous injury pathways*

Gene manipulation	Effect on cellular dysfunction	MCA occlusion	Effect on infarct size	Reference
Dnmt deletion	reduced DNA methylation	transient	decrease	Endres *et al* 2000 [18]
PS (presenilin)1 inactivation	perturbed calcium homeostasis	transient	increase	Mattson *et al* 2000 [55]
APP (amyloid precursor protein) overexpression	increased APP synthesis	permanent	increase	Zhang *et al* 1997 [80]
AGN (angiotensinogen) deletion	vasodilation	permanent	decrease	Maeda *et al* 1999 [49]
PCA2 (phospholipase A2) deletion	reduced arachidonic acid release	transient	decrease	Bonventre *et al* 1997 [4]

Conclusions

The use of genetically modified animals for the dissection of complex molecular injury cascades is a valuable addition to the repertoire of experimental stroke research. Important insights obtained by this approach are the differentiation between the dual role of NO for injury evolution, depending on the origin of generation [14], and the elucidation of the importance of free radical scavenging systems for minimizing tissue injury after ischemia-reperfusion [8]. Other investigations contributed to the identification of various putative molecular modulators of cell death. However, as ischemic injury in genetically modified animals may be influenced both by differences in genetic background and by various methodological influences, interpretations may be biased by prior knowledge, particularly when conflicting results are obtained. It is also disappointing that to the present no common molecular target for therapeutical interventions has been established in different experimental models of ischemia. This may reflect the multimodality of ischemic injury but it can also be interpreted as the failure of molecular stroke research to identify a key regulator of ischemic or post-ischemic survival. However, whatever this regulator may be, genetically modified animals will be of considerable importance to test its relevance under various conditions of ischemic injury.

Acknowledgment

This investigation was supported by EC grant QLG3-CT-2000-00934.

References

1. Aoki Y, Huang ZH, Thomas SS, Bhide PG, Huang I, Moskowitz MA, Reeves SA (2000) Increased susceptibility to ischemia-induced brain damage in transgenic mice overexpressing a dominant negative form of SHP2. FASEB J 14: 1965–1973
2. Asahi M, Asahi K, Jung JC, Zoppo GJd, Fini ME, Lo EH (2000) Role for matrix metalloproteinase 9 after focal cerebral ischemia: Effects of gene knockout and enzyme inhibition with BB-94. J Cereb Blood Flow Metab 20: 1681–1689
3. Bilbao Fd, Guarin E, Nef P, Vallet P, Giannakopoulos P, Dubois-Dauphin M (2000) Cell death is prevented in thalamic fields but not in injured neocortical areas after permanent focal ischaemia in mice overexpressing the anti-apoptotic protein Bcl-2. Eur J Neurosci 12: 921–934
4. Bonventre JV, Huang ZH, Taheri MR, Oleary E, Li E, Moskowitz MA, Sapirstein A (1997) Reduced fertility and postischaemic brain injury in mice deficient in cytosolic phospholipase A(2). Nature 390: 622–625
5. Bruce AJ, Boling W, Kindy MS, Peschon J, Kraemer PJ, Carpenter MK, Holtsberg FW, Mattson MP (1996) Altered neuronal and microglial responses to excitotoxic and ischemic brain injury in mice lacking TNF receptors. Nat Med 2: 788–794
6. Brusa R (1999) Genetically modified mice in neuropharmacology. Pharmacol Res 39: 405–419
7. Campagne MV, Thibodeaux H, van Bruggen N, Cairns B, Gerlai R, Palmer JT, Williams SP, Lowe DG (1999) Evidence for a protective role of metallothionein-1 in focal cerebral ischemia. Proc Nat Acad Sci USA 96: 12870–12875
8. Chan PH (2001) Reactive oxygen radicals in signaling and damage in the ischemic brain. J Cereb Blood Flow Metab 21: 2–14
9. Chan PH, Kamii H, Yang GY, Gafni J, Epstein CJ, Carlson E, Reola L (1993) Brain infarction is not reduced in SOD-1 transgenic mice after a permanent focal cerebral ischemia. NeuroReport 5: 293–296
10. Chen JF, Huang ZH, Ma JY, Zhu JM, Moratalla R, Standaert D, Moskowitz MA, Fink JS, Schwarzschild MA (1999) A(2a) adenosine receptor deficiency attenuates brain injury induced by transient focal ischemia in mice. J Neurosci 19: 9192–9200
11. Clark WM, Rinker LG, Lessov NS, Hazel K, Hill JK, Stenzel-Poore M, Eckenstein F (2000) Lack of interleukin-6 expression is not protective against focal central nervous system ischemia. Stroke 31: 1715–1720
12. Connolly ES, Winfree CJ, Stern DM, Solomon RA, Pinsky DJ (1996) Procedural and strain-related variables significantly affect outcome in a murine model of focal cerebral ischemia. Neurosurgery 38: 523–531
13. Crumrine RC, Thomas AL, Morgan PF (1994) Attenuation of p53 expression protects against focal ischemic damage in transgenic mice. J Cereb Blood Flow Metab 14: 887–891
14. Dalkara T, Yoshida T, Irikura K, Moskowitz MA (1994) Dual role of nitric oxide in focal cerebral ischemia. Neuropharmacology 33: 1447–1452
15. Dirnagl U, Iadecola C, Moskowitz MA (1999) Pathobiology of ischaemic stroke: an integrated view. Trends Neurosci 22: 391–397
16. Eliasson MJL, Huang ZH, Ferrante RJ, Sasamata M, Molliver ME, Snyder SH, Moskowitz MA (1999) Neuronal nitric oxide synthase activation and peroxynitrite formation in ischemic stroke linked to neural damage. J Neurosci 19: 5910–5918
17. Eliasson MJL, Sampei K, Mandir AS, Hurn PD, Traystman RJ, Bao J, Pieper A, Wang ZQ, Dawson TM, Snyder SH, Dawson VL (1997) Poly(ADP-ribose) polymerase gene disruption renders mice resistant to cerebral ischemia. Nat Med 3: 1089–1095
18. Endres M, Meisel A, Biniszkiewicz D, Namura S, Prass K, Ruscher K, Lipski A, Jaenisch R, Moskowitz MA, Dirnagl U (2000) DNA methyltransferase contributes to delayed ischemic brain injury. J Neurosci 20: 3175–3181
19. Ferriero DM, Holtzman DM, Black SM, Sheldon RA (1996) Neonatal mice lacking neuronal nitric oxide synthase are less vulnerable to hypoxic-ischemic injury. Neurobiol Dis 3: 64–71
20. Friedlander RM, Gagliardini V, Hara H, Fink KB, Li WW, Macdonald G, Fishman MC, Greenberg AH, Moskowitz MA, Yuan JY (1997) Expression of a dominant negative mutant of interleukin-1-beta converting enzyme in transgenic mice prevents neuronal cell death induced by trophic factor withdrawal and ischemic brain injury. J Exp Med 185: 933–940
21. Fujii M, Hara H, Meng W, Vonsattel JP, Huang ZH, Moskowitz MA (1997) Strain-related differences in susceptibility to transient forebrain ischemia in SV129 and C57Black/6 mice. Stroke 28: 1805–1810
22. Fujimura M, Morita-Fujimura Y, Kawase M, Copin J-C, Calagui B, Epstein CJ, Chan PH (1999) Manganese superoxide dismutase mediates the early release of mitochondrial cytochrome c and subsequent DNA fragmentation after permanent focal cerebral ischemia in mice. J Neurosci 19: 3414–3422
23. Gordon JW, Harold G, Leila Y (1993) Transgenic animal methodologies and their applications. Human Cell 6: 161–169
24. Grilli M, Barbieri I, Basudev H, Brusa R, Casati C, Lozza G, Ongini E (2000) Interleukin-10 modulates neuronal threshold of vulnerability to ischaemic damage. Eur J Neurosci 12: 2265–2272
25. Grotta J (1995) Why do all drugs work in animals but none in stroke patients? 2. Neuroprotective therapy. J Inter Med 237: 89–94
26. Guo ZH, Kindy MS, Kruman I, Mattson MP (2000) Als-linked Cu/Zn-SOD mutation impairs cerebral synaptic glucose and glutamate transport and exacerbates ischemic brain injury. J Cereb Blood Flow Metab 20: 463–468
27. Hara H, Fink K, Endres M, Friedlander RM, Gagliardini V, Yuan J, Moskowitz MA (1997) Attenuation of transient focal cerebral ischemic injury in transgenic mice expressing a mutant ICE inhibitory protein. J Cereb Blood Flow Metab 17: 370–375
28. Hara H, Huang PL, Panahian N, Fishman MC, Moskowitz MA (1996) Reduced brain edema and infarction volume in mice lacking the neuronal isoform of nitric oxide synthase after transient MCA occlusion. J Cereb Blood Flow Metab 16: 605–611
29. Hata R, Gass P, Mies G, Wiessner C, Hossmann K-A (1998) Attenuated c-fos mRNA induction after middle cerebral artery occlusion in CREB knockout mice does not modulate focal ischemic injury. J Cereb Blood Flow Metab 18: 1325–1335
30. Hata R, Gillardon F, Michaelidis TM, Hossmann K-A (1999) Targeted disruption of the bcl-2 gene in mice exacerbates focal ischemic brain injury. Metabolic Brain Dis 14: 117–124

31. Hata R, Maeda K, Hermann D, Mies G, Hossmann K-A (2000) Dynamics of regional brain metabolism and gene expression after middle cerebral artery occlusion in mice. J Cereb Blood Flow Metab 20: 306–315
32. Hata R, Maeda K, Hermann D, Mies G, Hossmann K-A (2000) Evolution of brain infarction after transient focal cerebral ischemia in mice. J Cereb Blood Flow Metab 20: 937–946
33. Hata R, Mies G, Wiessner C, Fritze K, Hesselbarth D, Brinker G, Hossmann K-A (1998) A reproducible model of middle cerebral artery occlusion in mice – hemodynamic, biochemical, and magnetic resonance imaging. J Cereb Blood Flow Metab 18: 367–375
34. Holschneider DP, Scremin OU, Huynh L, Chen K, Shih JC (1999) Lack of protection from ischemic injury of monoamine oxidase B-deficient mice following middle cerebral artery occlusion. Neurosci Lett 259: 161–164
35. Hossmann K-A (1994) Viability thresholds and the penumbra of focal ischemia. Ann Neurol 36: 557–565
36. Huang ZH, Huang PL, Ma JY, Meng W, Ayata C, Fishman MC, Moskowitz MA (1996) Enlarged infarcts in endothelial nitric oxide synthase knockout mice are attenuated by nitro-L-arginine. J Cereb Blood Flow Metab 16: 981–987
37. Huang ZH, Huang PL, Panahian N, Dalkara T, Fishman MC, Moskowitz MA (1994) Effects of cerebral ischemia in mice deficient in neuronal nitric oxide synthase. Science 265: 1883–1885
38. Iadecola C, Zhang FY, Casey R, Nagayama M, Rose ME (1997) Delayed reduction of ischemic brain injury and neurological deficits in mice lacking the inducible nitric oxide synthase gene. J Neurosci 17: 9157–9164
39. Kadotani H, Namura S, Katsuura G, Terashima T, Kikuchi H (1998) Attenuation of focal cerebral infarct in mice lacking NMDA receptor subunit NR2C. NeuroReport 9: 471–475
40. Keller JN, Kindy MS, Holtsberg FW, StClair DK, Yen HC, Germeyer A, Steiner SM, Brucekeller AJ, Hutchins JB, Mattson MP (1998) Mitochondrial manganese superoxide dismutase prevents neural apoptosis and reduces ischemic brain injury: suppression of peroxynitrite production, lipid peroxidation, and mitochondrial dysfunction. J Neurosci 18: 687–697
41. Kinouchi H, Epstein CJ, Mizui T, Carlson E, Chen SF, Chan PH (1991) Attenuation of focal cerebral ischemic injury in transgenic mice overexpressing CuZn superoxide dismutase. Proc Nat Acad Sci USA 88: 11158–11162
42. Kitagawa K, Matsumoto M, Mabuchi T, Yagita Y, Ohtsuki T, Hori M, Yanagihara T (1998) Deficiency of intercellular adhesion molecule 1 attenuates microcirculatory disturbance and infarction size in focal cerebral ischemia. J Cereb Blood Flow Metab 18: 1336–1345
43. Kondo T, Reaume AG, Huang TT, Carlson E, Murakami K, Chen SF, Hoffman EK, Scott RW, Epstein CJ, Chan PH (1997) Reduction of CuZn-superoxide dismutase activity exacerbates neuronal cell injury and edema formation after transient focal cerebral ischemia. J Neurosci 17: 4180–4189
44. Lawrence MS, Ho DY, Sun GH, Steinberg GK, Sapolsky RM (1996) Overexpression of bcl-2 with herpes simplex virus vectors protects CNS neurons against neurological insults in vitro and in vivo. J Neurosci 16: 486–496
45. Le D, Das SY, Wang YF, Yoshizawa T, Sasaki YF, Takasu M, Nemes A, Mendelsohn M, Dikkes P, Lipton SA, Nakanishi N (1997) Enhanced neuronal death from focal ischemia in AMPA-receptor transgenic mice. Mol Brain Res 52: 235–241
46. Lo EH, Hara H, Rogowska J, Trocha M, Pierce AR, Huang PL, Fishman MC, Wolf GL, Moskowitz MA (1996) Temporal correlation mapping analysis of the hemodynamic penumbra in mutant mice deficient in endothelial nitric oxide synthase gene expression. Stroke 27: 1381–1385
47. Lukkarinen JA, Grohn OHJ, Alhonen LI, Janne J, Kauppinen RA (1999) Enhanced ornithine decarboxylase activity is associated with attenuated rate of damage evolution and reduction of infarct volume in transient middle cerebral artery occlusion in the rat. Brain Res 826: 325–329
48. MacManus JP, Koch CJ, Jian M, Walker T, Zurakowski B (1999) Decreased brain infarct following focal ischemia in mice lacking the transcription factor E2F1. NeuroReport 10: 2711–2714
49. Maeda K, Hata R, Bader M, Walther T, Hossmann K-A (1999) Larger anastomoses in angiotensinogen-knockout mice attenuate early metabolic disturbances after middle cerebral artery occlusion. J Cereb Blood Flow Metab 19: 1092–1098
50. Maeda K, Hata R, Gillardon F, Hossmann K-A (2001) Aggravation of brain injury after transient focal ischemia in p53 deficient mice. Molecular Brain Research 88: 54–61
51. Maeda K, Hata R, Hossmann K-A (1998) Differences in the cerebrovascular anatomy of C57Black/6 and SV129 mice. NeuroReport 9: 1317–1319
52. Maeda K, Hata R, Hossmann K-A (1999) Regional metabolic disturbances and cerebrovascular anatomy after permanent middle cerebral artery occlusion in C57Black/6 and SV129 mice. Neurobiol Dis 6: 101–108
53. Martinou JC, Dubois-Dauphin M, Staple JK, Rodrigues I, Frankowski H, Missotten M, Albertini P, Talabot D, Catsicas S, Pietra C, Huarte J (1994) Overexpression of BCL-2 in transgenic mice protects neurons from naturally occurring cell death and experimental ischemia. Neuron 13: 1017–1030
54. Mattson MP, Culmsee C, Yu ZF (2000) Apoptotic and antiapoptotic mechanisms in stroke. Cell Tissue Res 301: 173–187
55. Mattson MP, Zhu HY, Yu J, Kindy MS (2000) Presenilin-1 mutation increases neuronal vulnerability to focal ischemia in vivo and to hypoxia and glucose deprivation in cell culture: involvement of perturbed calcium homeostasis. J Neurosci 20: 1358–1364
56. Morikawa E, Mori H, Kiyama Y, Mishina M, Asano T, Kirino T (1998) Attenuation of focal ischemic brain injury in mice deficient in the epsilon1 (NR2A) subunit of NMDA receptor. J Neurosci 18: 9727–9732
57. Nagai N, Mol Md, Lijnen HR, Carmeliet P, Collen D (1999) Role of plasminogen system components in focal cerebral ischemic infarction. A gene targeting and gene transfer study in mice. Circulation 99: 2440–2444
58. Nagayama M, Aber T, Nagayama T, Ross ME, Iadecola C (1999) Age-dependent increase in ischemic brain injury in wild-type mice and in mice lacking the inducible nitric oxide synthase gene. J Cereb Blood Flow Metab 19: 661–666
59. Panahian N, Yoshiura M, Maines MD (1999) Overexpression of heme oxygenase-1 is neuroprotective in a model of permanent middle cerebral artery occlusion in transgenic mice. J Neurochem 72: 1187–1203
60. Paschen W, Olah L, Mies G (2000) Effect of transient focal ischemia of mouse brain on energy state and NAD levels: No evidence that NAD depletion plays a major role in secondary disturbances of energy metabolism. J Neurochem 75: 1675–1680
61. Pieper AA, Blackshaw S, Clements EE, Brat DJ, Krug DK, White AJ, Pinto-Garcia P, Favit A, Conover JR, Snyder SH, Verma A (2000) Poly(ADP-ribosyl)ation basally activated by DNA strand breaks reflects glutamate-nitric oxide neurotransmission. Proc Nat Acad Sci USA 97: 1845–1850
62. Rajdev S, Hara K, Kokubo Y, Mestril R, Dillmann W, Weinstein PR, Sharp FR (2000) Mice overexpressing rat heat shock protein 70 are protected against cerebral infarction. Ann Neurol 47: 782–791

63. Rosenbaum DM, Gupta G, D'Amore J, Singh M, Weidenheim K, Zhang H, Kessler JA (2000) Fas (CD95/APO-1) plays a role in the pathophysiology of focal cerebral ischemia. J Neurosci Res 61: 686–692
64. Sampei K, Goto S, Alkayed NJ, Crain BJ, Korach KS, Traystman RJ, Demas GE, Nelson RJ, Hurn PD (2000) Stroke in estrogen receptor-alpha-deficient mice. Stroke 31: 738–743
65. Schauwecker PE, Steward O (1997) Genetic determinants of susceptibility to excitotoxic cell death: Implications for gene targeting approaches. Proc Natl Acad Sci USA 94: 4103–4108
66. Schielke GP, Yang GY, Shivers BD, Betz AL (1998) Reduced ischemic brain injury in interleukin-1-beta converting enzyme-deficient mice. J Cereb Blood Flow Metab 18: 180–185
67. Schneider A, Martin-Villalba A, Weih F, Vogel J, Wirth T, Schwaninger M (1999) NF-kappa B is activated and promotes cell death in focal cerebral ischemia. Nat Med 5: 554–559
68. Sharp FR (1998) Stress genes protect brain. Ann Neuro 44: 581–583
69. Sheng H, Bart RD, Oury TD, Pearlstein RD, Crapo JD, Warner DS (1999) Mice overexpressing extracellular superoxide dismutase have increased resistance to focal cerebral ischemia. Neuroscience 88: 185–191
70. Soriano SG, Coxon A, Wang YF, Frosch MP, Lipton SA, Hickey PR, Mayadas TN (1999) Mice deficient in MAC-1 (CD11B/CD18) are less susceptible to cerebral ischemia/reperfusion injury. Stroke 30: 134–139
71. Soriano SG, Lipton SA, Wang YMF, Xiao M, Springer TA, Gutierrez-Ramos JC, Hickey PR (1996) Intercellular adhesion molecule-1-deficient mice are less susceptible to cerebral ischemia – reperfusion injury. Ann Neurol 39: 618–624
72. Tabrizi P, Wang L, Seeds N, McComb JG, Yamada S, Griffin JH, Carmeliet P, Weiss MH, Zlokovic BV (1999) Tissue plasminogen activator (tPa) deficiency exacerbates cerebrovascular fibrin deposition and brain injury in a murine stroke model. Studies in tPa-deficient mice and wild-type mice on a matched genetic background. Arterioscl Thromb Vasc Biol 19: 2801–2806
73. Takagi Y, Mitsui A, Nishiyama A, Nozaki K, Sono H, Gon Y, Hashimoto N, Yodoi J (1999) Overexpression of thioredoxin in transgenic mice attenuates focal ischemic brain damage. Proc Nat Acad Sci USA 96: 4131–4136
74. Thomas KR, Capecchi MR (1987) Site-directed mutagenesis by gene targeting in mouse embryo-derived stem cells. Cell 51: 503–512
75. Walder CE, Green SP, Darbonne WC, Mathias J, Rae J, Dinauer MC, Curnutte JT, Thomas GR (1997) Ischemic stroke injury is reduced in mice lacking a functional NADPH oxidase. Stroke 28: 2252–2258
76. Wang YMF, Tsirka SE, Strickland S, Stieg PE, Soriano SG, Lipton SA (1998) Tissue plasminogen activator (tPA) increases neuronal damage after focal cerebral ischemia in wild-type and tPA-deficient mice. Nat Med 4: 228–231
77. Weisbrot-Lefkowitz M, Reuhl K, Perry B, Cahn PH, Inouye M, Mirochnitchenko O (1998) Overexpression of human glutathione peroxidase protects transgenic mice against focal cerebral ischemia/reperfusion damage. Mol Brain Res 53: 333–338
78. Wiessner C, Allegrini PR, Rupalla K, Sauer D, Oltersdorf T, McGregor AL, Bischoff S, Böttiger BW, Putten Hvd (1999) Neuron-specific transgene expression of Bcl-X_L but not Bcl-2 genes reduced lesion size after permanent middle cerebral artery occlusion in mice. Neurosci Lett 268: 119–122
79. Yang GY, Schielke GP, Gong C, Mao Y, Ge HL, Liu XH, Betz AL (1999) Expression of tumor necrosis factor-alpha and intercellular adhesion molecule-1 after focal cerebral ischemia in interleukin-1 beta converting enzyme deficient mice. J Cereb Blood Flow Metab 19: 1109–1117
80. Zhang FY, Eckman C, Younkin S, Hsiao KK, Iadecola C (1997) Increased susceptibility to ischemic brain damage in transgenic mice overexpressing the amyloid precursor protein. J Neurosci 17: 7655–7661
81. Zhao X, Haensel C, Araki E, Ross ME, Iadecola C (2000) Gene-dosing effect and persistence of reduction in ischemic brain injury in mice lacking inducible nitric oxide synthase. Brain Res 872: 215–218

Correspondence: Prof. Dr. K.-A. Hossmann, Max-Planck-Institute for Neurological Research, Department of Experimental Neurology, Gleueler Str. 50, D-50931 Cologne, Germany. e-mail: Hossmann@mpin-koeln.mpg.de

Progress in the understanding of brain injury from ischemia

Acta Neurochir (2004) [Suppl] 89: 49–54

Printed in Austria

The Janus face of inflammation in ischemic brain injury

X. Wang and **G. Z. Feuerstein**

Department of Cardiovascular Disease Research, DuPont Pharmaceuticals Company, Wilmington, Delaware, USA

Summary

Brain ischemia elicits an intense inflammatory reaction as evidenced by endogenous activation of microglia and infiltration of leukocytes from the systemic circulation into the brain. A key issue regarding the well-described inflammation in brain injury is whether this reaction is of salutary or detrimental nature in the short and longterm post ischemia. In this brief review, evidence in support for the possible beneficial as well as detrimental role of inflammatory cells and mediators in ischemic brain injury is highlighted. We offer the opinion that both benefits and adverse effects of the inflammatory reaction at large depent on the levels of a specific mediator, the temporal relationships to the injury, the context in which the mediator operates and the spatial relationships to the injury.

Keywords: Inflammation; brain ischemia; brain injury; therapeutics.

Stroke is the third cause of death in most developed countries and the leading cause of cardiovascular death in Japan and China. Stroke management is a leading health burden in all developed countries considering loss of productive years and rehabilitation costs. Epidemiological studies conducted over the past 10 years consistently demonstrate steady reduction in the incidence of stroke in developed countries until the very recent years where the incidence seems to plateau [3, 5]. This remarkable reduction in the incidence of strokes is attributed not to successful treatment of acute stroke but improved preventive messures, including (i) effective management of risk factors such as hypertension and diabetes, (ii) prevention of thromboembolic events with anti-coagulant treatment, (coumadin for chronic atrial fibrillation) and antiplatelet agents (aspirin, clopidogrel) for primary and secondary prevention, (iii) reduction of atherosclerosis burden by lipid lowering agents and physical activity, and (iv) better understanding of environmental, psychological (stress) and behavioral (smoking and dietary habits) factors. In fact, effective treatment of hypertension, smoking cessation and anti-coagulation alone has been estimated to prevent ~75% of stroke events in the USA.

While the incidence of stroke has declined steadily over the past decades, progress in treatment of acute stroke has been disappointing. At the turn of the 21st century, management of patients with acute stroke is still largely conservative, featuring clinical assessment, preservation of vital function and elimination of obvious causes such as emboli and hemodynamic factors. Only minority of patients with acute ischemic stroke benefit from specific therapy with thrombolytics (~2–5%) since the therapeutic window is limited to (3 hours post onset of stroke) due to major adverse events (in particular, intracerebral hemorrhage). In only one area of stroke management, diagnosis, substantial progress has been made consequent to the remarkable progress in imaging techniques that better assess the nature and location of the ischemic event [6, 13, 14].

The failure of the medical and pharmaceutical community to provide improved management for acute stroke patients is in particular striking in view of the enormous resources that have been applied to invent, develop and apply new therapeutics for stroke. The clinical trials conducted over the past decade by various pharmaceutical houses have explored the efficacy of various agents that have been intensely researched in many experimental paradigms that feature components of the human stroke condition. Yet, none of the clinical trials conducted with neuroprotective agents resulted in benefits to the patients. This disappointing reality has raised many questions regarding the schemes and strategies that underwrote the pharmaceutical development of drugs for stroke. In this re-

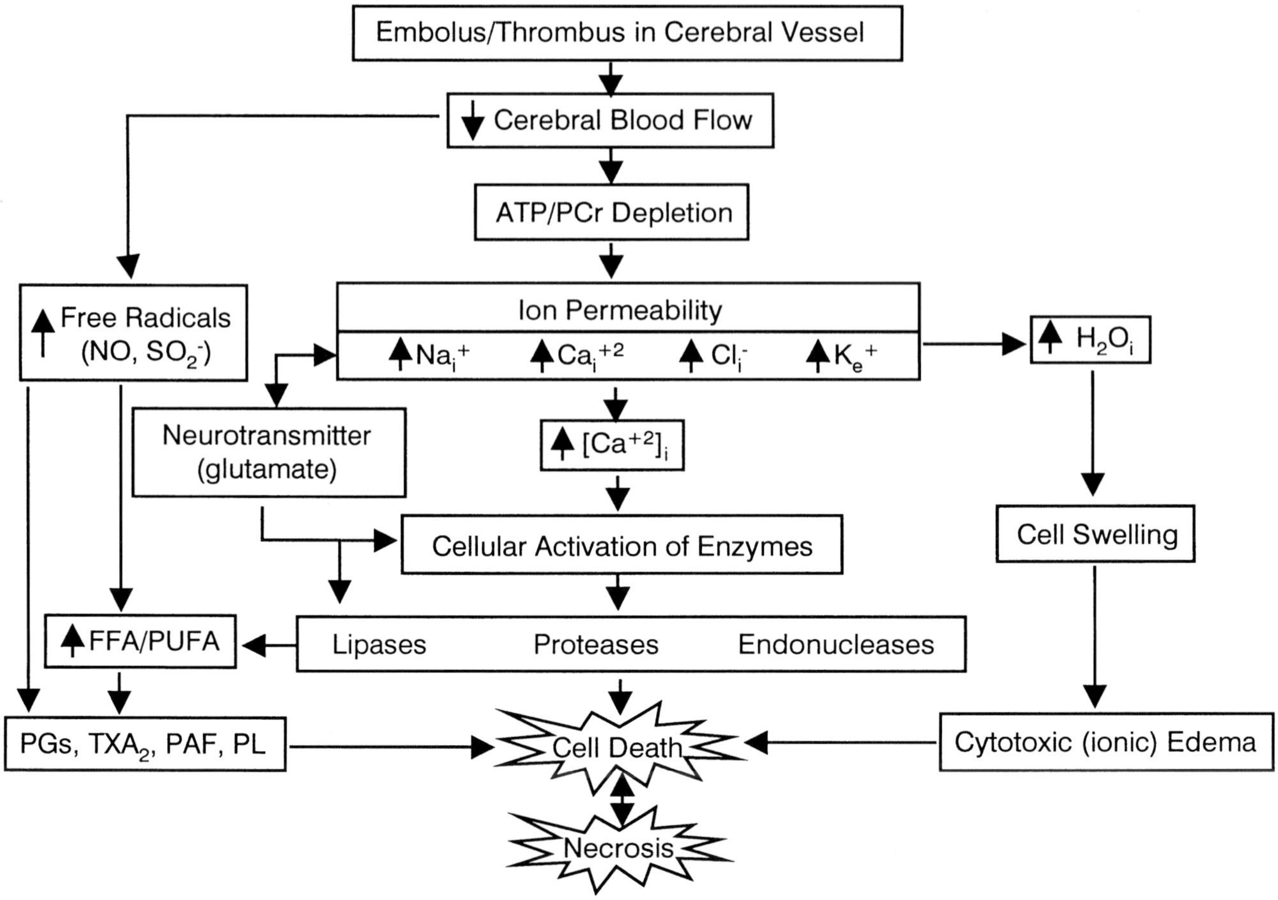

Fig. 1. Schematic diagram illustrating changes occurring in thromboembolic cerebral ischemia that contribute to loss of cellular integrity and tissue destruction/infarction

gard, one of the most pressing issue is whether the molecular targets that have been chosen for manipulation by the agents that failed in the trials were indeed the proper ones. Inspection of the compounds that have been used in phase III studies suggest that so far, inhibitors and antagonists of excitotoxic neurotransmitters such as glutamate and its co-activators, glycine, have not produced the expected benefits. Other targets such as adhesion molecule (ICAM-1), ion channels (Ca^{+2}, Na^{+}) and oxygen radicals have not as yet demonstrated efficacy either. The reasons for the choices of these targets, largely based on research in the 1970–1980s, is depicted in figure 1 where pathways of neuronal damage are shown. Figure 1, a highly simplified representation of the enormously complex perturbations of brain neurochemistry by ischemia, focuses on 3 major molecular pathways: (i) The accumulation of Na^{+}/Ca^{+2} ions consequent to loss of membrane potential and unregulated ion fluxes; (ii) massive release of neurotransmitters that are excitotoxic – of which glutamate was held as the 'primary suspect' and (iii) oxidative stress that leads to radical formations, lipid peroxidation and indiscriminate membrane and organelle damage. However, as shown in Fig. 2, the *time frame* for activation and action of the molecular targets that failed in clinical trials is likely to be a major reason that these pharmacological agents failed in clinical development. Figure 2 provides temporal perspective to this issue; clearly, at the time of patients availability for treatment in a medical facility (usually beyond 3 hours after the onset of the ischemic event) the early biochemical events that result from loss of membrane potential-ion fluxes, excitotoxic mediator release and radical formation, have long exercised their effect. Several hours after the ischemic attack, new molecular and biochemical events are emerging which include *de novo* gene expression, protein synthesis and cellular events not seen

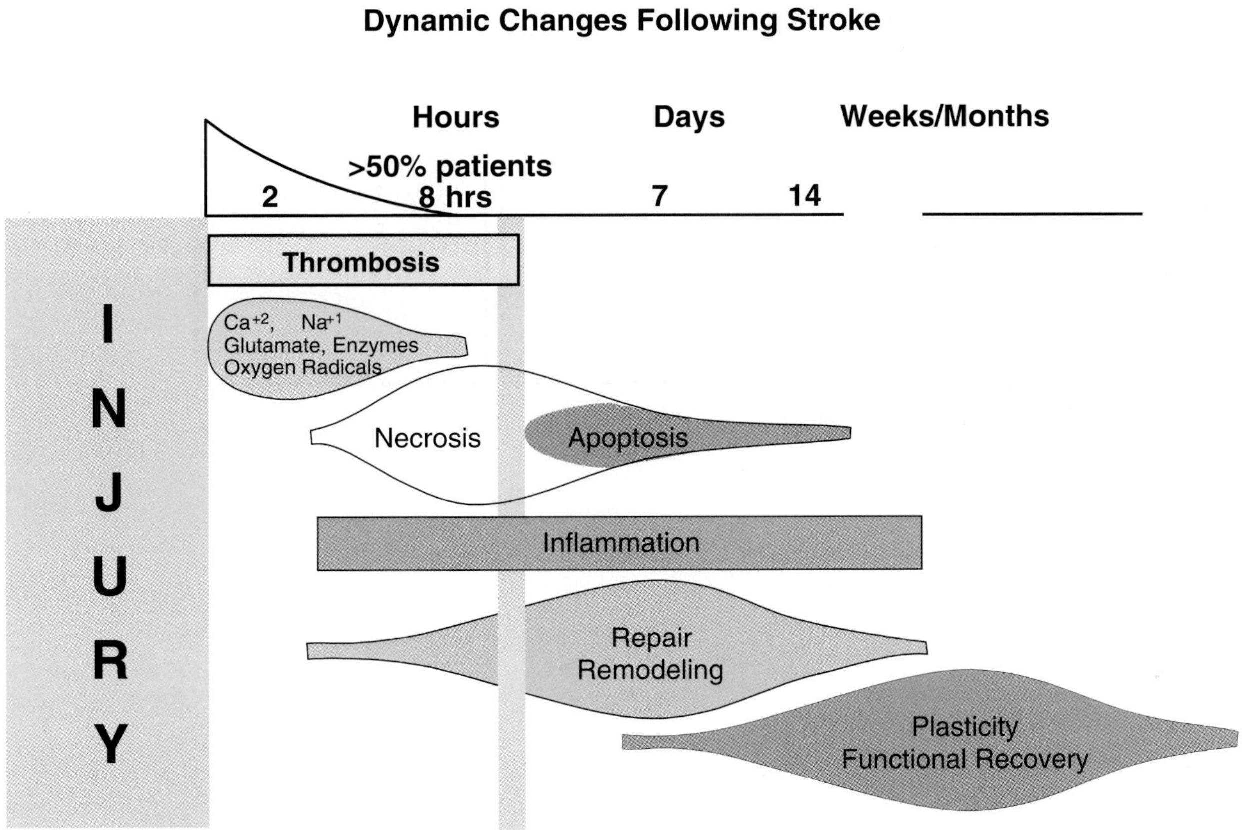

Fig. 2. Schematic diagram depicts the dynamic changes following ischemic stroke

in the normal healthy brain tissue. These cellular components include activation of microglia and infiltration of blood borne leukocytes across the blood brain barrier into the brain. In brief, an acute inflammatory reaction is initiated few hours after brain ischemia that lasts for several days has been launched. At that time, brain cells commence on extensive transcription and translation of genes that express inflammatory mediators such as cytokines and chemokines, highly conducive inflammatory milieu in the ischemic region (Fig. 3).

The inflammatory reaction induced by an ischemic challenge to brain tissue has been well-documented in experimental as well as clinical studies. Over the past decade, stroke researchers inspecting brain tissue following various time points after stroke, observed indisputably inflammatory cells (neutrophils, monocytes) at the site of injury. With the aid of highly specific molecular, biochemical and immunohistochemical techniques, the presence of numerous inflammatory mediators in and around the ischemic brain tissue has been documented. In brief, the presence of 'inflammatory' cytokines, interleukins, chemokines, leukocytes – endothelial adhesion molecules, etc., triggered intense research on strategies to abolish the emergence and/or effects of these mediators. It is important, however, to keep in mind that the inflammatory reaction at large is designed as a defense mechanism against invading toxic organisms and noxious agents as well as providing for 'tissue cleansing' and repair. This fundamental role of the inflammatory reaction in preserving tissue health poses the issue of whether or not inflammatory cells and mediators that are present in the injured brain are 'friend or foe'. The basic research literature on this subject is replete with reports on 'wrong doing' of inflammatory mediators and 'beneficial' effect of 'suppressors' of its components such as leukocyte depletion, adhesion molecule antagonists (ICAM-1, E- or P-selectins), anti-cytokines and interleukin antagonists. A minority of critical reports has been largely ignored. However, careful inspection of the data regarding the det-

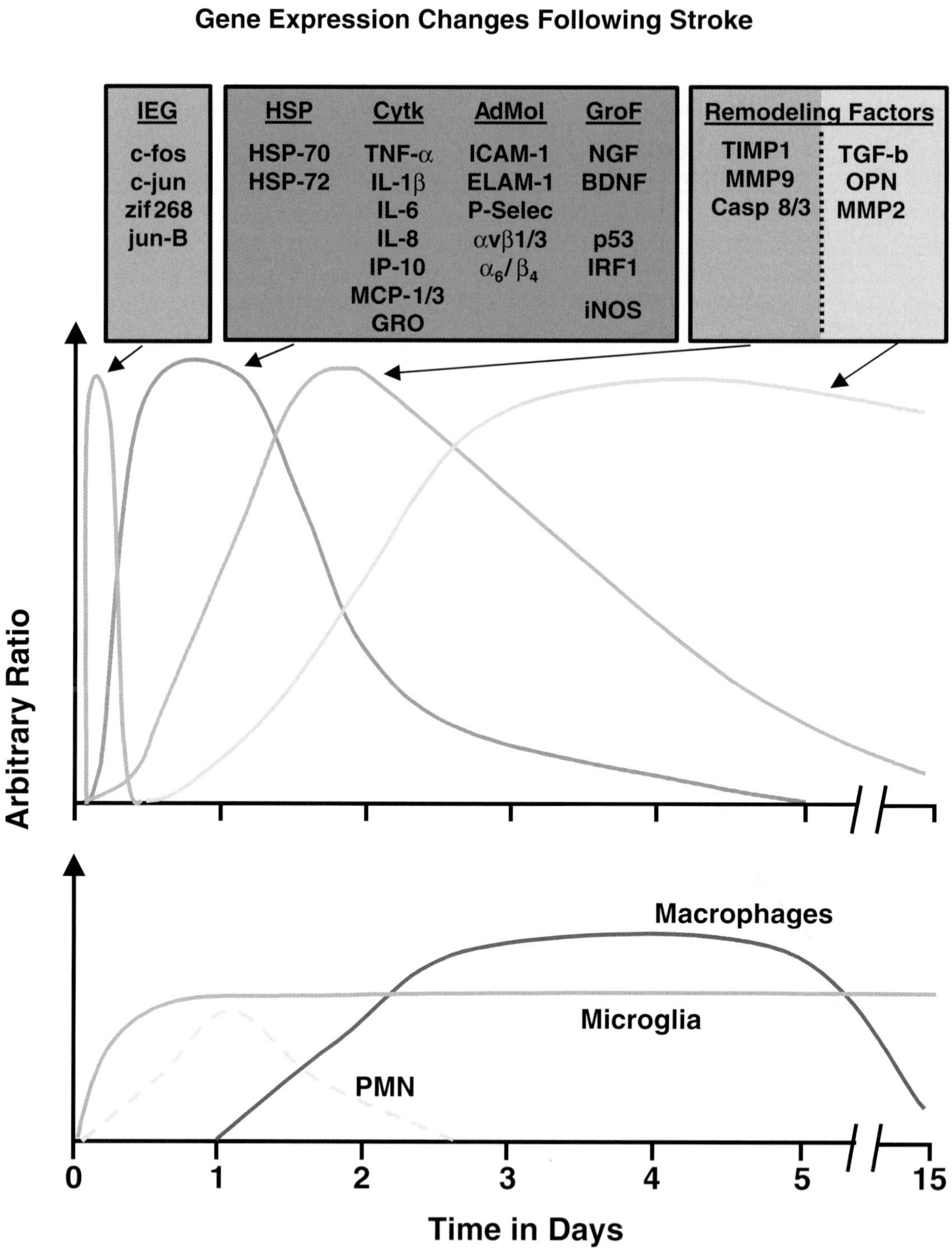

Fig. 3. Gene expression in rat ischemic cortex after middle cerebral artery occlusion. Four waves of ischemic gene expression include early response genes/transcription factors *(wave 1)*, heat shock proteins, pro-inflammatory mediators and growth factors *(wave 2)*, proteinases and proteinase inhibitors *(wave 3)* and delayed remodeling proteins *(wave 4)*. The leukocyte wave, including early polymorphonuclear *(PMN)* neutrophils and later monocytes/macrophages infiltration, as well as activated microglia, is illustrated in the lower panel. Astrocyte activation (gliosis) occurs following leukocyte infiltration in the ischemic brain tissue

rimental role of inflammation in stroke reveals the following potential pitfalls:

1. Pharmacological studies where inflammatory mediators are injected acutely into the brain (normal or ischemic) could be quite artificial; the doses may be unrealistic in respect to the endogenous production and release capacity. In addition, correlation between the levels of these inflammatory mediators and the spatial and temporal context to the disease condition have often been ignored.
2. Transgenic animal models where discrete deletion of certain cytokine or cytokine receptor genes (the 'bad guys') were subjected to brain ischemia, have shown more extensive injury and inferior long-term recovery over the wild type mice – an opposite result than the expected: 'protection'. Most notable are the TNFα −/− mice where deletion of the cytokine or the cytokine receptors resulted in significantly larger necrotic tissue and poor functional outcome; so also for IL-6 −/− mice [1, 9, 11].
3. Cytokines have a 'reputation' of pro-inflammatory function, yet some cytokines such as IL-10 have been shown to possess neuroprotective efficacy in various models of brain injury including stroke [10]. In fact, even TNFα and IL-1β, two cytokines most often cited as detrimental in the context of stroke, have been shown to provide neuroprotection and in fact, condition brain tissue into a state of 'tolerance' to ischemic insults when administered before the onset of the ischemic insult [7, 12].
4. While activated macrophages are viewed as villains when spotted in the brain, the growth promoting and neuroprotective potential of factors released from activated macrophages has been grossly overlooked. This is evidenced by remarkable recovery induced by application of homologous activated macrophages to injured spinal cord in rats [8]. In addition, studies where MBP (myelin basic protein)-activated T-cell have been applied to injured optic nerves show neuroprotection to the retina [5], an unexpected result based on the 'known' role of MBP-activated T-cells in white matter injury that is associated with multiple sclerosis.
5. From the clinical perspective, it is well established that glucocorticoids, the most potent and fast acting anti-inflammatory drugs known to medicine, are of no therapeutic benefits in stroke patients [4]. Likewise, none of the common non-steroidal anti-inflammatory agents (NSAIDs, e.g., aspirin, indomethacin, ibuprofen, etc.) have proven beneficial in the acute treatment of stroke.
6. Most recently, clinical trials in acute stroke patients with the anti-intercellular adhesion molecule-1 (ICAM-1) antibody have been terminated following futility analysis [2]. In fact, a trend towards adverse outcome was noted. While the cause for this situation remains to be analyzed, the failure of the ICAM-1 trials in stroke is consistent with lack of efficacy of broad (steroids) or more specific (NSAID) spectrum of anti-inflammatory agents in treatment of stroke.

In summary, it is important to call for more careful analysis of the role of inflammation in ischemic brain injury. Special emphasis was placed on the diverse biological and pathological aspects of inflammation and the potential for salutary as well as detrimental components of this reaction. It is hoped that further research on the role of inflammatory mediators will lead to new strategies and formulas for novel preventive and therapeutic measures in stroke.

References

1. Bruce AJ, Boling W, Kindy MS *et al* (1996) Altered neuronal and microglial responses to excitotoxic and ischemic brain injury in mice lacking TNF receptors. Nature Med 2: 788–794
2. DeGraba TJ (1998) The role of inflammation after acute stroke: utility of pursuing anti-adhesion molecule therapy. Neurology 51(S3): S62–S68
3. Heart and Stroke Statistical Update, American Heart Association (1999)
4. Millikan CH, McDowell F, Easton JD (1987) Stroke, chapter 8. Lea & Febiger, Philadelphia, pp 117–130
5. Moalem G, Leibowitz-Amit R, Yoles E, Mor F, Cohen IR, Schwartz M (1999) Autoimmune T cells protect neurons from secondary degeneration after central nervous system axotomy. Nature Med 5: 49–63
6. Neumann-Haefelin T, Moseley ME, Albers GW (2000) New magnetic resonance imaging methods for cerebrovascular disease: emerging clinical applications. Ann Neurol 47: 559–570
7. Ohtsuki T, Ruetzler CA, Tasaki K, Hallenbeck JM (1996) Interleukin-1 mediates induction of tolerance to global ischemia in gerbil hippocampal CA1 neurons. J Cereb Blood Flow Metab 16: 1137–1142
8. Rapalino O, Lazarov-Spiegeler O, Agranov E *et al* (1998) Implantation of stimulated homologous macrophages results in partial recovery of paraplegic rats. Nature Med 4: 814–821
9. Schrebel U, Raghupath R, Nakamura M *et al* (1999) Differential acute and chronic responses of tumor necrosis factor – deficient mice to experimental brain injury. Proc Natl Acad Sci USA 96: 8721–8726
10. Spera PA, Ellison JA, Feuerstein GZ, Barone FC (1998) IL-10 reduces rat brain injury following focal stroke. Neurosci Lett 251: 189–192

11. Stahel PF, Shohami E, Younis FM *et al* (2000) Experimental closed head injury: analysis of neurological outcome, blood brain Barrier, dysfunction, intracranial neutrophil infiltration, and neuronal cell death in mice deficient in genes for pro-inflammatory cytokines. J Cerebral Blood flow Metab 20: 369–380
12. Tasaki K, Ruetzler CA, Ohtsuki T, Martin D, Nawashiro H, Hallenbeck JM (1997) Lipopolysaccharide pre-treatment induces resistance against focal cerebral ischemic damage in spontaneously hypertensive rats. Brain Res 748: 267–270
13. Tong DC, Albers GW (2000) Diffusion and perfusion magnetic resonance imaging for the evaluation of acute stroke: potential use in guiding thrombolytic therapy. Curr Opin Neurol 13: 45–50
14. Wityk RJ, Beauchamp NJ Jr (2000) Diagnostic evaluation of stroke. Neurol Clin 18: 357–378
15. Wolf PA, Kannel, D'Agostino WB (1998) Epidemiology of stroke. In: Cerebrovascular disease: pathophysiology, diagnosis and management. In: Ginsberg MD, Bogousslavsky J (eds) Blackwell Science, USA, pp 834–849

Correspondence: Giora Z. Feuerstein, M.D., Department of Cardiovascular Sciences Dupont Pharmaceuticals Company, Experimental Station, E400/3257A, Wilmington, DE 19880-0400, USA. e-mail: giora.z.feuerstein@dupontpharma.com

Acta Neurochir (2004) [Suppl] 89: 55–61

Printed in Austria

The natural course of lesion development in brain ischemia

T. Back[1] and **O. G. Schüler**[2]

[1] Department of Neurology, Philipps University Marburg, Marburg, Germany
[2] Department of Neurology, Ludwig-Maximilians University Munich, Munich, Germany

Summary

Histopathologic and NMR imaging studies show that focally ischemic brain lesions tend to increase in size over time. In animal models of stroke as well as in patients presenting with hemispheric stroke, considerable lesion growth was observed. In focal cerebral ischemia, lesions predominantly enlarge early (<12 hrs postinsult) and show complete ischemic injury due to pan necrosis in the vast majority of affected tissue. In global cerebral ischemia – a condition that is present after cardiac arrest – lesions appear late (>12 hrs) in selectively vulnerable brain regions and neurons are damaged by apoptosis. The short resuscitation time of the brain explains why periods of global ischemia result in widespread and global loss of energy metabolites combined with diffuse brain edema and global damage. Mechanisms involved in lesion growth include excitotoxicity, peri-infarct depolarizations, lactacidosis, microcirculatory disturbances, and flow-metabolism uncoupling among others. Problems involved in the subject under focus are related to maturation phenomena of injury and the different imaging modalities (metabolic imaging, NMR imaging, positron emission tomography) that require a subtly differentiated interpretation of the alterations observed.

Keywords: Ischemia; NMR imaging; cardiac arrest; stroke.

Introduction

Non-invasive methods like NMR imaging and positron emission tomography (PET) have stimulated observations on the behaviour of ischemic lesions with regard to their temporal and spatial dynamics. Surprisingly, territorial brain infarcts tend to enlarge during an ongoing period of ischemia; this has been shown in animal models of stroke [24, 25, 34] and in the clinical setting. Almost half of the patients who presented with acute hemispheric stroke showed a marked increase in lesion size by >20% occurring over the initial 7 days poststroke [10]. The situation is less clear in global cerebral ischemia, a condition that differs in many pathophysiologic aspects from focal ischemia. In animal experiments, global ischemia may either lead to recovery or to secondary deterioration of the tissue status associated with global reduction of energy metabolites [31]. However, the time course of changes in the brain parenchyma of patients with cardiac arrest is not well documented [2] and is difficult to assess due to the patchy nature of lesions that tend to be subtle. The purpose of this review is to describe the dynamics of lesion development both in focal and global cerebral ischemia. Comparisons between experiments and clinical data are drawn. The potential mechanisms of those processes are discussed and finally, the problems involved in the matter are described to direct future research in the field.

States of focal brain ischemia

In focal ischemia, the growth of lesions has been investigated by using histopathologic studies [20, 21]. These studies demonstrated the phenomenon of infarct maturation, i.e., that there is time needed for the macroscopic and microscopic changes to become apparent on histological sections of the brain. At least 2–3 hours following the ischemic impact are necessary for the cells to show distinct ischemic changes such as generalized swelling, shrinkage and scalloping of neurons and the formation of vacuoles in dendrites [21]. During this period, it is difficult to assess the lesion size using histological means because the ischemic changes are sparse and not well demarcated at the borders towards non-affected tissue. About 6–12 hrs after onset of ischemia, typical features appear that indicate irreversible tissue damage such as axonal swelling, so-called 'red neurons', and the occurrence of neuronal and astrocytic 'ghost cells'. Based on those pathologic findings it is suggested to differentiate early lesion growth

(<12 hrs postocclusion) from late one (>12 hrs postocclusion). This anticipates that at later stages of the process of infarction morphologic alterations seem to be irreversible in contrast to very early changes such as astrocytic swelling with otherwise normal appearing neuropil and preserved neurons.

Histopathological studies by Garcia and co-workers [21] have demonstrated in the rat middle cerebral artery (MCA) occlusion model that the ischemic area covered 10% of the hemisphere at 1-h, 22% at 2-h, 38% at 6-h and 50% at 12-h postocclusion. Thereafter, lesion growth slowed considerably or ceased altogether. The mathematical function of growth describes a rising asymptotic curve that approximates a certain maximum lesion volume. It may be assumed, however, that the values given for the initial 3 hours do not reflect the real ischemic impact on the tissue under focus as shown later in this review. The predominant type of cell death in models of permanent MCA occlusion is pannecrosis. It has to be mentioned that in models of reversible MCA occlusion and – to a quite restricted amount – also in permanent vessel occlusion some cells die from apoptosis that only occurs if the energy state of tissue is grossly maintained [37, 38].

The regional distribution of ATP or glucose is another marker of ischemic lesions that is more reliable in the very early stage of infarction compared to histopathology. In permanent vessel occlusion models it has been shown that areas with grossly reduced ATP/glucose are significantly enlarged during the initial 2 hrs following MCA occlusion [34]. In this study, ATP reduction covered 22% of the ischemic hemisphere at 30 min and 50% at 2 hrs. This considerable magnitude of lesion enlargement was also demonstrated for other variables, i.e., areas with solid acidosis (61% at 30 min; 70% at 2 hrs postocclusion) or regions that exhibit a disturbance of diffusion as measured by NMR diffusion imaging (54% at 30 min; 67% at 2 hrs postocclusion) [24, 25, 34]. Interestingly, the alterations of ATP content, glucose content, tissue pH or tissue diffusion all were dependent on distinct thresholds of cerebral blood flow (CBF). It is important to note that the measurement of the apparent diffusion coefficient (ADC) only showed a reduction if CBF went lower than 0.34 ml/g/min (30-min ischemia) or 0.41 ml/g/min (2-h ischemia), respectively [34]. This means that with ongoing ischemia, the CBF thresholds for certain pathologic processes (ATP reduction, acidosis, diffusion disturbance) increase and are a function of time. It also makes clear that the change in the diffusion signal occurs at CBF rates that would alter the electrical function of the brain, i.e., correspond to the upper threshold of the ischemic penumbra [3], but not necessarily lead to morphologic damage.

Our measurements of CBF show that in the infarct core of the enlarging brain lesion, the actual CBF values tend to decrease with ongoing ischemia time (from 0.25 ml/g/min at 30 min to 0.10 ml/g/min at 2 hrs postocclusion) [34]. The increasing disturbance of microcirculation in the central part of the lesions has been also observed by other investigators [19, 26] and is attributed to accumulation of lactate and microscopic cell swelling that hinders blood flow in the capillary bed. The enlargement of the ischemic territory seems to occur at the expense of the ischemic penumbra: while the penumbra becomes restricted to a rim in the periphery of the evolving infarct, the infarct core area spreads from the lesion center to more peripheral regions, thereby occupying formerly penumbral areas. The comparison between histologic sections, images of metabolism (ATP, glucose, lactate, tissue pH) and diffusion-weighted images (DWI) at 7 hrs after onset of ischemia shows that now nearly congruent areas are observed that display overt infarction, ATP loss or disturbed diffusion, respectively [6]. Interestingly, there are also regions outside the ischemic lesion that exhibit clearly increased levels of lactate – a metabolite that may increase viscosity in the microcirculation and accounts, by part, for the marked acidosis in flow-compromised areas. Longitudinal studies that employ NMR diffusion imaging are capable to document lesion evolution over time even in individual animals that suffer from stroke. Figure 1 presents such an example in which the increase in affected tissue is visible on repeated DWI, but also the increase in signal intensity (brightness of the lesion center) over time.

Recently, the development of ischemic lesion volume by using repeated diffusion imaging was demonstrated in a model of clot embolism of the MCA in rats [14]. Compared to the lesion volume at 30-min, final lesion size at 8-h postocclusion had increased by ~70%. In experiments with transient vessel obstruction, the lesion growth, as visualized on DWI, can be reversed if the brain is reperfused within 1 h postocclusion [40]. Regions like the putamen and, depending on the stroke model, temporal parts of the cortex show consistent infarction. With ongoing ischemia, predominantly cortical areas are recruited into the process of lesion growth.

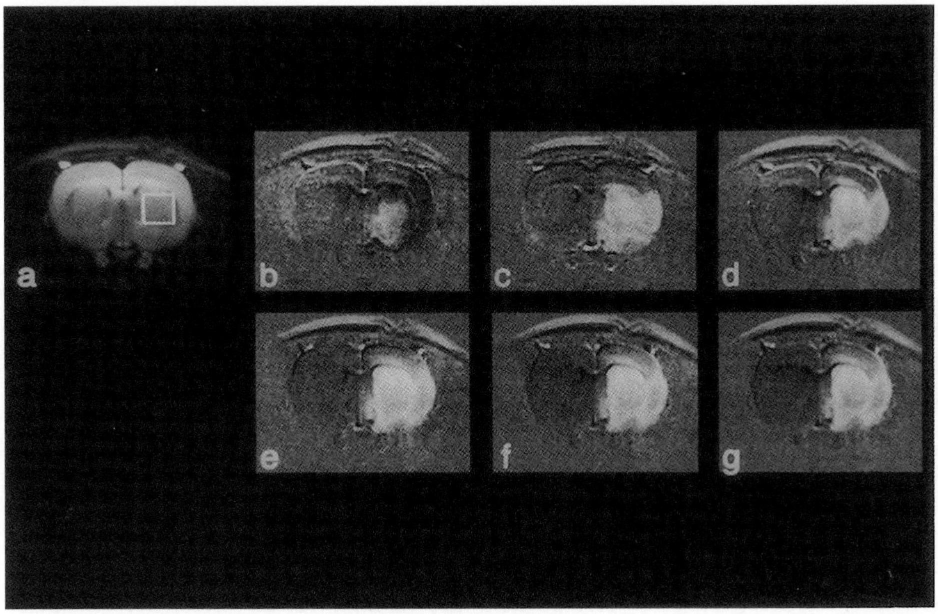

Fig. 1. Lesion development in experimental MCA occlusion in rat measured by repeated NMR diffusion-weighted imaging. Left top: Control condition (a) in a coronal brain slice. Images (b) to (g): Repeated measurements of diffusion-weighted images (subtraction images) equally distributed over a 6-hours period postocclusion. Note the lesion growth and the increase in signal intensity within the lesion. (Courtesy M. Hoehn, Cologne)

In human stroke, a very similar pattern has been observed by various investigators [10, 11, 33]. About 50% of hemispheric territory infarcts tend to increase in size over the first days poststroke. The magnitude of mean infarct progression varied from 48% up to 97% [10, 11, 33, 43]. Progression of lesions could be predicted if the initial investigation would show a large perfusion deficit in bolus-tracking perfusion maps that would clearly encompass the tissue with an altered diffusion signal [33]. This finding has been interpreted in a sense that the perfusion-diffusion mismatch area (perfusion reduced, diffusion normal) would represent – at least by part – the ischemic penumbra that obviously in most cases undergoes a secondary deterioration over time. This interpretation is conceivable, but difficult to prove as long as the NMR perfusion maps do not measure CBF in quantitative terms. Currently, it remains unclear to which extent those areas suffer from critical hypoperfusion [43]. However, the progressive metabolic derangement of periinfarct tissue has been documented by serial PET measurements of CBF, glucose and oxygen metabolism in a cohort of acute stroke patients [28]. We know from angiographic studies in man that the outcome of patients presenting with large hemispheric perfusion deficits is grossly dependent on the collateral supply via the anterior/posterior communicating arteries, pial anastomoses and other variable arteries connecting the territories of the external and internal carotid artery. There is also sound evidence that infarct progression can be reversed by early reperfusion that can be promoted by thrombolytic agents such as tissue plasminogen activator (TPA) [18, 19, 35]. Thus, subareas of the ischemic lesions can be salvaged by reperfusion or TPA-associated recanalization as already shown in rat models of MCA occlusion [19, 40]. Figure 2 shows a speculative synposis of metabolic and imaging information in various subareas of a human brain territory infarct. The onion-shaped structure of such lesions with regard to the CBF and ADC gradients gradually decreasing from normal-appearing surrounding tissue towards the ischemic infarct core has been shown in experimental stroke [30] as well as in acute human stroke [5]. It is likely that the outer layers of the ischemic lesion that have comparably higher flow values compared to the infarct core may benefit from reperfusion or – in the future – from neuroprotective strategies. They may represent ischemic subareas that, during the process of lesion enlargement, have been last recruited into the lesion area. It is, however, unlikely, that any of the centrally located areas that are supplied by functional end arteries (for example, the

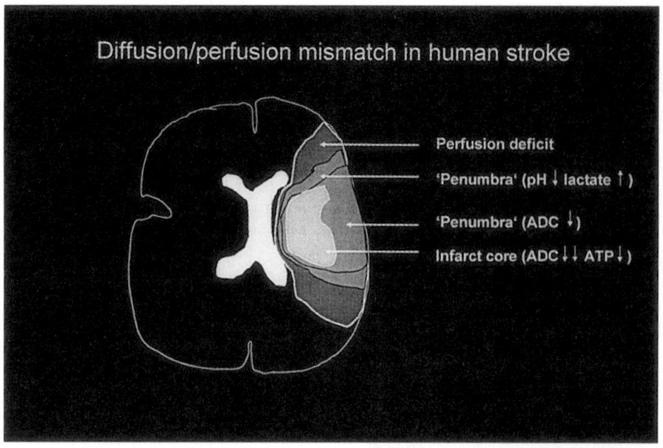

Fig. 2. Diffusion/perfusion mismatch in human stroke (speculative synopsis). ADC: apparent diffusion coefficient

lentiform nucleus) could recover by any given therapy. Heiss and colleagues have shown that the degree of initial critical hypoperfusion (as measured by PET) well predicted the final infarct size. In their stroke patients, the critically perfused brain volume amounted to 15 ml (measured < 3 hrs after symptom onset) whereas after 2–3 weeks the final infarct volume was 22 ml encompassing the initial perfusion deficit [29]. Whether or not this pattern of infarct evolution also applies to other stroke types such as hemodynamic or small vessel occlusive infarcts, currently remains unanswered. Lesion progression has been reported in a case of lacunar infarction, recently [49]; systematic studies are lacking.

States of global brain ischemia

Much less is known about the temporal and spatial dynamics of lesions in global ischemia/anoxia. Studies by Hossmann and coworkers [31] show that prolonged gobal ischemia often results in secondary deterioration during the reperfusion phase that, in those animals, leads to depletion of energy metabolites, sound acidosis and a dramatic increase in lactate content. In some animals, however, recovery can be observed that is mainly dependent on successful reperfusion. This pathologic condition that imitates cardiac arrest in man, results in a rapid (< 10 min) and marked (68% of control) decrease in the ADC when measured by repeated NMR diffusion imaging. If we apply the lesion assessment as used in focal ischemia, one would estimate a nearly 100% lesion size after 1-h of global ischemia (visible already after the initial 10 min) that may or may not resolve during a 180-min reperfusion period. A classical finding in other models of global ischemia, e.g., the four-vessel-occlusion model in rats [47], is a circumscribed damage to the CA1 sector of the hippocampal formation that appears after 3 days. The number of dead CA1 neurons has been shown to increase from 3 to 7 days post insult [13]. Other predilective regions prone to injury in global ischemia are the thalamus, the basal ganglia and the cortical layers 3 to 5. Due to the subtlety of histopathologic changes that consist mainly of selective neuronal injury of the delayed type, it is difficult to assess lesion size in quantitative terms. In the literature, we do not find solid numbers for affected volumes of this process. The preferred type of cell death in this condition is apoptosis, and not necrosis as seen in focal ischemia [13, 44].

The morphological and imaging data on cardiac arrest patients are rare [2, 12, 23]. Recently, Arbaelez *et al.* published NMR findings in a series of patients with global cerebral ischemia following cardiac arrest [2]. It becomes obvious that DWI are capable of depicting ischemic/anoxic tissue changes in the acute and early subacute phase (up to 14 days post insult) that were not displayed on T1- or T2-weighted images or, alternatively, seen at a later stage of the disease [2]. There are no systematic longitudinal studies available to answer the question of cerebral lesion growth in human cardiac arrest. However, there is sound clinical evidence that longer durations of global circulatory arrest exceeding the resuscitation time of ≈10 min, almost uniformly result in fatal outcome with generalized brain edema, obscuration of gray-white matter junctions and widespread laminar necrosis of the cortex.

Mechanisms of injury

A variety of potential causes for lesion development (studied mainly in focal cerebral ischemia) are discussed and include: (i) the time-dependent increase in microcirculatory flow disturbances [34], (ii) the occurrence of severe lactacidosis in the infarct core [6, 7], (iii) the occurrence of spreading depression-like phenomena in the periinfact area [8, 15, 41], (iv) the time-dependent increase in the glucose utilization/blood flow uncoupling in the infarct border [9, 42], and (v) other molecular responses such as the occurrence of apoptosis and inflammatory changes [17, 37, 38, 44].

In experimental stroke, irregular depolarizations occur in the surroundings of an ischemic focus that travel over the cortex like spreading depression of electrical activity [8, 36, 41]. The number of such peri-infarct depolarizations (PIDs) correlated with final infarct size [4, 39] and could be effectively blocked by glutamate anatagonists or initiation of recanalization that both reduced infarct volume [32, 45, 48]. By using repetitive NMR diffusion imaging, the propagation of the ischemic lesion which is dependent on the occurrence of PIDs, has been demonstrated in a rat model of stroke [15, 46]. A recent attempt to measure similar changes in ADC that resemble PIDs in acute human stroke, was unsuccessful [5]. PIDs are closely related to a well-established concept of ischemic tissue injury, namely the excitotoxicity concept [16]. The high number of glutamate receptors on the surface of cortical neurons but also in other parts of the brain explain that glutamate release may overstimulate those neurons due to impaired clearance mechanisms for excitotoxic transmitters. Other factors that contribute to lesion growth are related to the progressive impairment of CBF and the associated derangement of glucose and energy metabolism. A striking uncoupling between near-to-normal glucose utilization in the presence of compromised flow has been demonstrated in animal models of stroke [9, 22, 42]. It seems unlikely that any tissue could survive this mismatch between energy demand and blood flow supply on longer terms.

Another important pathophysiologic factor is the excess generation of lactate due to the initiation of anaerobic metabolism. The lactate spreads over large parts of the affected hemisphere and – together with hydrogen ions from ATP hydrolysis – contributes to the severe acidosis that may further damage neurons [7]. Apart from these acute metabolic changes, molecular responses like the upregulation of immediate-early genes, the formation of stress proteins, the upregulation of pro-apoptotic proteins and inflammatory changes occur that may modulate the final ischemic injury in the subacute phase. However, it is very unlikely that this modulation would account for changes in lesion volume that exceed the 5 or 10% limit [29].

Potential pitfalls

Problems involved in the topic under focus are related to the maturation phenomenon of infarct histology as described in the section on focal ischemia. In global ischemia, histological changes may be too subtle for valid volume assessment. During the course of ischemia, the occurrence of brain edema complicates the volume estimation of ischemic lesions because the entire affected hemisphere (still including non-affected tissue) may be swollen and enlarged compared to the contralateral side. In the chronic stage of infarction, tissue shrinkage occurs that, in contrast, may result in underestimation of the affected volume of brain parenchyma. It has to be mentioned that the occurrence of scattered neuronal loss in the periinfarct zones accounts for up to 15% of the total ischemic injury volume [1, 4] and, thus, complicates lesion quantification. The study of infarct development and lesion evolution requires a methodology that enables longitudinal studies. New modalities of NMR imaging appear to be the most promising tool for this type of study. Repeated PET studies of CBF and glucose/oxygen metabolism are an alternative that has been applied successfully in animal stroke and human studies [27, 28]. However, attention has to be paid to the fact that the ischemic lesions, as visible on NMR diffusion images, may differ in size from areas with reduced energy metabolites, from areas with severe perfusion deficits or from regions with decreased glucose consumption as determined by PET or autoradiography, respectively.

Acknowledgement

The support of one of the authors (T.B.) by the Wicker Foundation, Bad Wildungen, is gratefully acknowledged.

References

1. Alexis NE, Back T, Zhao W, Dietrich WD, Watson BD, Ginsberg MD (1996) Neuro-behavioral consequences of induced spreading depression following photothrombotic middle cerebral artery occlusion. Brain Res 706: 273–282
2. Arbelaez A, Castillo M, Mukherji SK (1999) Diffusion-weighted MR imaging of global cerebral anoxia. Am J Neuroradiol 20: 999–1007
3. Astrup J, Siesjö BK, Symon L (1981) Thresholds in cerebral ischemia – The ischemic penumbra. Stroke 12: 723–725
4. Back T, Ginsberg MD, Dietrich WD, Watson BD (1996) Induction of spreading depression in the ischemic hemisphere following experimental middle cerebral artery occlusion: Effect on infarct morphology. J Cereb Blood Flow Metab 16: 202–213
5. Back T, Hirsch JG, Szabo K, Gass A (2000) Failure to demonstrate peri-infarct depolarizations by repetitive MR diffusion imaging in acute human stroke. Stroke 31: 2901–2906
6. Back T, Hoehn-Berlage M, Kohno K, Hossmann K-A (1994) Diffusion NMR imaging in experimental stroke: correlation with cerebral metabolites. Stroke 25: 494–500
7. Back T, Hoehn M, Mies G, Busch E, Schmitz B, Kohno K, Hossmann KA (2000) Penumbral tissue alkalosis in focal cerebral ischemia: relationship to energy metabolism, blood flow, and steady potential. Ann Neurol 47: 485–492

8. Back T, Kohno K, Hossmann K-A (1994) Cortical negative DC deflections following middle cerebral artery occlusion and KCl-induced spreading depression: Effect on blood flow, tissue oxygenation and electroencephalogram. J Cereb Blood Flow Metab 14: 12–19
9. Back T, Zhao W, Ginsberg MD (1995) Three-dimensional image analysis of brain glucose metabolism/blood flow uncoupling and its electrophysiological correlates in the acute ischemic penumbra following middle cerebral artery occlusion. J Cereb Blood Flow Metab 15: 566–577
10. Baird AE, Benfield A, Schlaug G, Siewert B, Lövblad K-O, Edelman RR, Warach S (1997) Enlargement of human cerebral ischemic lesion volumes measured by diffusion-weighted magnetic resonance imaging. Ann Neurol 41: 581–589
11. Barber PA, Darby DG, Desmond PM, Yang Q, Gerraty RP, Jolley D, Donnan GA, Tress BM, Davis SM (1998) Prediction of stroke outcome with echoplanar perfusion- and diffusion-weighted MRI. Neurology 51: 418–426
12. Berek K, Lechleitner P, Luef G, Felber S, Saltuari L, Schinnerl A, Traweger C, Dienstl F, Aichner F (1995) Early determination of neurological outcome after prehospital cardiopulmonary resuscitation. Stroke 26: 543–549
13. Bottiger BW, Schmitz B, Wiessner C, Vogel P, Hossmann KA (1998) Neuronal stress response and neuronal cell damage after cardiocirculatory arrest in rats. J Cereb Blood Flow Metab 18: 1077–1087
14. Brinker G, Franke C, Hoehn M, Uhlenkuken U, Hossmann KA (1999) Thrombolysis of cerebral clot embolism in rat: effect of treatment delay. NeuroReport 10: 3269–3272
15. Busch E, Gyngell M, Eis M, Hoehn-Berlage M, Hossmann K-A (1996) Potassium-induced cortical spreading depression during focal cerebral ischemia in rats: contribution to lesion growth assessed by diffusion-weighted NMR and biochemical imaging. J Cereb Blood Flow Metab 16: 1090–1099
16. Choi DW (1992) Excitotoxic cell death. J Neurobiol 23: 1261–1276
17. Clark RK, Lee EV, Fish CJ, White RF, Price WJ, Jonak ZL, Feuerstein GZ, Barone FC (1993) Development of tissue damage, inflammation and resolution following stroke: an immunohistochemical and quantitative planimetric study. Brain Res Bull 31: 565–572
18. del Zoppo GJ, Higashida RT, Furlan AJ, Pessin MS, Rowley HA, Gent M (1998) PROACT: a phase II randomized trial of recombinant pro-urokinase by direct arterial delivery in acute middle cerebral artery stroke. PROACT Investigators. Prolyse in acute cerebral thromboembolism. Stroke 29: 4–11
19. Franke C, Brinker G, Pillekamp F, Hoehn M (2000) Probability of metabolic tissue recovery after thrombolytic treatment of experimental stroke: a magnetic resonance spectroscopic imaging study in rat brain. J Cereb Blood Flow Metab 20: 583–591
20. Garcia JH, Kamijyo Y (1974) Cerebral infarction evolution of histopathological changes after occlusion of the middle cerebral artery in primates. Exp Neurol 33: 408–421
21. Garcia JH, Yoshida Y, Chen H, Li Y, Zhang ZG, Lian J, Chen S, Chopp M (1993) Progression from ischemic injury to infarct following middle cerebral artery occlusion in the rat. Am J Pathol 142: 623–635
22. Ginsberg MD, Back T, Zhao W (1995) Three-dimensional metabolic and hemodynamic imaging of the normal and ischemic rat brain. Acta Neurochir (Wien) 66: 44–49
23. Grubb NR, Fox KA, Smith K, Best J, Blane A, Ebmeier KP, Glabus MF, O'Carroll RE (2000) Memory impairment in out-of-hospital cardiac arrest survivors is associated with global reduction in brain volume, not focal hippocampal injury. Stroke 31: 1509–1514
24. Gyngell M, Back T, Hoehn-Berlage M, Kohno K, Hossmann K-A (1994) Transient cell depolarization after permanent middle cerebral artery occlusion: An observation by diffusion-weighted MRI and localized 1H-MRS. Magn Reson Med 31: 337–341
25. Gyngell M, Busch E, Schmitz B, Kohno K, Back T, Hoehn-Berlage M, Hossmann K-A (1995) Evolution of acute focal cerebral ischaemia in rats observed by localised 1H-MRS, diffusion-weighted MRI, and electrophysiological monitoring. NMR Biomed 8: 206–214
26. Hakim AM, Hogan MJ, Carpenter S (1992) Time course of cerebral blood flow and histological outcome after focal cerebral ischemia in rats. Stroke 23: 1138–1143
27. Heiss W-D, Graf R, Wienhard K, Lottgen J, Saito R, Fujita T, Rosner G, Wagner R (1994) Dynamic penumbra demonstrated by sequential multitracer PET after middle cerebral artery occlusion in cats. J Cereb Blood Flow Metab 14: 892–902
28. Heiss W-D, Huber M, Fink GR, Herholz K, Pietrzyk U, Wagner R, Wienhard K (1992) Progressive derangement of periinfarct viable tissue in ischemic stroke. J Cereb Blood Flow Metab 12: 193–203
29. Heiss WD, Thiel A, Grond M, Graf R (1999) Contribution of immediate and delayed ischaemic damage to the volume of final infarcts. Lancet 353: 1677–1678
30. Hoehn-Berlage M, Norris DG, Kohno K, Mies G, Leibfritz D, Hossmann KA (1995) Evolution of regional changes in apparent diffusion coefficient during focal ischemia of rat brain: the relationship of quantitative diffusion NMR imaging to reduction in cerebral blood flow and metabolic disturbances. J Cereb Blood Flow Metab 15: 1002–1011
31. Hossmann KA, Fischer M, Bockhorst K, Hoehn-Berlage M (1994) NMR imaging of the apparent diffusion coefficient (ADC) for the evaluation of metabolic suppression and recovery after prolonged cerebral ischemia. J Cereb Blood Flow Metab 14: 723–731
32. Iijima T, Mies G, Hossmann K-A (1992) Repeated negative DC deflections in rat cortex following middle cerebral artery occlusion are abolished by MK-801: effect on volume of ischemic injury. J Cereb Blood Flow Metab 12: 727–733
33. Karonen JO, Vanninen RL, Liu Y, Ostergaard L, Kuikka JT, Nuutinen J, Vanninen EJ, Partanen PLK, Vainio PA, Korhonen K (1999) Combined diffusion and perfusion MRI with correlation to single-photon emission CT in acute ischemic stroke. Ischemic penumbra predicts infarct growth. Stroke 30: 1583–1590
34. Kohno K, Hoehn-Berlage M, Mies G, Back T, Hossmann K-A (1995) Relationship between diffusion-weighted magnetic resonance images, cerebral blood flow and energy state in experimental brain infarction. Magn Reson Imag 13: 73–80
35. Kummer Rv, Holle R, Rosin L, Forsting M, Hacke W (1995) Does arterial recanalization improve outcome in carotid territory stroke? Stroke 26: 581–587
36. Leao AAP (1944) Spreading depression of activity in the cerebral cortex. J Neurophysiol 7: 359–390
37. Li Y, Chopp M, Jiang N, Xao F, Zaloga C (1995) Temporal profile of in situ DNA fragmentation after transient middle cerebral artery occlusion in the rat. J Cereb Blood Flow Metab 15: 389–397
38. Linnik MD, Zobrist RH, Hatfield MD (1993) Evidence supporting a role for programmed cell death in focal cerebral ischemia in rats. Stroke 24: 2002–2009
39. Mies G, Iijima T, Hossmann K-A (1993) Correlation between periinfarct DC shifts and ischemic neuronal damage in rat. NeuroReport 4: 709–711

40. Minematsu K, Li L, Sotak CH, Davis MA, Fisher M (1992) Reversible focal ischemic injury demonstrated by diffusion-weighted MR imaging in rats. Stroke 23: 1304–1311
41. Nedergaard M, Astrup J (1986) Infarct rim: Effect of hyperglycemia on direct current potential and [14C]2-deoxyglucose phosphorylation. J Cereb Blood Flow Metab 6: 607–615
42. Nedergaard M, Gjedde A, Diemer NH (1986) Focal ischemia of the rat brain: autoradiographic determination of cerebral glucose utilization, glucose content, and blood flow. J Cereb Blood Flow Metab 6: 414–424
43. Neumann-Haefelin T, Wittsack HJ, Wenserski F, Siebler M, Seitz R, Mödder U, Freund H-J (1999) Diffusion- and perfusion-weighted MRI. The DWI/PWI mismatch region in acute stroke. Stroke 30: 1591–1597
44. Ouyang YB, Tan Y, Comb M, Liu CL, Martone ME, Siesjo BK, Hu BR (1999) Survival- and death-promoting events after transient cerebral ischemia: phosphorylation of Akt, release of cytochrome C and Activation of caspase-like proteases. J Cereb Blood Flow Metab 19: 1126–1135
45. Park CK, Nehls DG, Graham DI, Teasdale GM, McCulloch J (1988) The glutamate antagonist MK-801 reduces focal ischemic brain damage in the rat. Ann Neurol 24: 543–551
46. Roether J, de Crespigny A, D'Arceuil H, Iwai K, Moseley ME (1996) Recovery of apparent diffusion coefficient after ischemia-induced spreading depression relates to cerebral perfusion gradient. Stroke 27: 980–987
47. Schmidt-Kastner R, Paschen W, Ophoff BG, Hossmann KA (1989) A modified four-vessel occlusion model for inducing incomplete forebrain ischemia in rats. Stroke 20: 938–946
48. Schüler OG, Plesnila N, Otto D, Baethmann AJ, Back T (2001) Early thrombolysis inhibits peri-infarct depolarizations in embolic MCA occlusion. NeuroReport 12 (18): 3943–3946
49. Terai S, Hori T, Miake S, Tamaki K, Saishoji A (2000) Mechanism in progressive lacunar infarction: a case report with magnetic resonance imaging. Arch Neurol 57: 255–258

Correspondence: Prof. Dr. Tobias Back, Department of Neurology, Philipps-University Marburg, R-Bultmann-Str 8, 35039 Marburg, Germany. e-mail: back@staff.uni-marburg.de

Acta Neurochir (2004) [Suppl] 89: 63–66

Printed in Austria

Pharmacological preconditioning in global cerebral ischemia

A. M. Brambrink, H. Noga, A. Astheimer, A. Heimann, and **O. Kempski**

Institut of Neurosurgical Pathophysiology, Johannes Gutenberg-University, Mainz, Germany

Summary

Single dose 3-nitropropionic acid (3-NPA) 24 hr before global ischemia improves neuronal survival in both, neocortex and hippocampus ('chemical preconditioning'). Neuronal survival after transient global ischemia requires new protein synthesis during recovery, especially of those with anti-apoptotic function. Bcl-2-protein is expressed in neurons that survive cerebral ischemia and may parallel the time course of tolerance after ischemic preconditioning. With this study we examined whether differences in bcl-2-protein expression compared to baseline may be involved in the induction of ischemic tolerance using 3-NPA.

Male Wistar rats received either a single intraperitoneal (i.p.) dose of 3-NPA (20 mg/kg), and were observed for 3 ($n = 4$), 12 ($n = 5$) or 24 hours ($n = 5$) or the same amount of vehicle and were observed for 24 h ($n = 8$, controls). Immunohistochemistry allowed to compare the intensity of bcl-2 immunoreactivity at three subsequent time points in hippocampus, dentate gyrus and parietal neocortex with that of control animals.

A single dose of 3-NPA caused a significant increase of bcl-2 protein immunoreactivity in hippocampal neurons, i.e. CA 1 (5 out of 5 animals, $p = 0.003$), CA 3 (5/5, $p = 0.003$), CA 4 (4/5, $p = 0.025$), and neocortex (5/5, $p = 0.004$), in a time dependent manner over a period of 24 hr after injection. Neuronal bcl-2 protein expression in CA 2 and dentate gyrus remained unchanged.

The data suggest a possible role of bcl-2-protein in chemical induction of ischemic tolerance using a single subtoxic dose of 3-NPA. Bcl-2-protein expression may be initiated by increased levels of reactive oxygen species (ROS) after 3-NPA administration, as shown by others. Additional bcl-2 protein may then be available to (1) control postischemic ROS burst, (2) protect the mitochondrial membranes, and (3) inhibit pro-apoptotic mechanisms.

Keywords: Tolerance induction, preconditioning, 3-NPA, bcl-2.

Introduction

Recently we showed in rats that moderate metabolic inhibition using 3-nitropropionic acid (3-NPA) improved neuronal survival after global ischemia as compared to control animals [17]. The effect has been termed "chemical preconditioning". Tolerance against ischemia was also observed in gerbil hippocampus after 3-NPA injection [21] and in ex-vivo experiments using rat hippocampal slices [18]. Various stress stimuli to neuronal tissue have been shown to be accompanied by increased levels of reactive oxygen species (ROS, oxidative stress) [6, 10, 13, 14, 19] and it has been suggested that ROS formation could represent an important initial step for the induction of ischemic tolerance in the brain [12, 22, 23]. However, further downstream effects remain unclear.

Neuronal survival after transient global ischemia depends in part on new protein synthesis during recovery, especially of those related to apoptosis repressor genes [5, 24]. Bcl-2-protein is present in neurons that survive global and focal ischemia and some authors suggested that the expression of bcl-2 protein may parallel the time course of tolerance after ischemic preconditioning [20].

With this study we therefore examined whether an enhanced bcl-2-protein expression is involved in chemical induction of tolerance to global cerebral ischemia by pretreatment with 3-NPA.

Methods

Male Wistar rats were randomly assigned to four different groups. Three groups of animals received a single intraperitoneal (i.p.) dose of 3-NPA (20 mg/kg), and were observed for 3 ($n = 4$), 12 ($n = 5$) or 24 hours ($n = 5$), respectively. The fourth group of animals was injected with the same amount of vehicle and was observed for 24 h ($n = 8$) serving as controls ("baseline").

At appropriate times brains were transcardially perfusion fixed, processed for paraffin embedding and sliced into coronal sections. Immunohistochemistry, including two cycles of microwave radiation, was performed using rabbit polyclonal antibody against bcl-2-protein (Santa Cruz Biotechnology Inc., USA).

Using the Optimas imaging system (Stemmer, Germany), the intensity of bcl-2 immunoreactivity in different regions of hippocampus, dentate gyrus and parietal neocortex was compared to control animals by three different investigators (AMB, AA, HN). Additionally, all brain sections were evaluated for morphologic evidence of neuronal cell damage.

Changes in immunoreactivity compared to baseline were expressed as 'animals per group' which showed an enhanced bcl-2 protein expression. Time dependent differences between groups were assessed by multiple logistic regression, using SigmaStat-2.0 routines (Jandel, Erkrath, Germany). Differences were considered as statistically significant at $p < 0.05$.

Results

A single application of 3-NPA (20 mg/kg, i.p.) resulted in increased bcl-2 protein immunoreactivity in neurons of hippocampus and neocortex in a time dependent manner over a period of 24 hr after injection. Figure 1 shows photomicrographs of representative animals. At baseline (vehicle treatment) neuronal immunoreactivity for bcl-2 protein was faint in CA1, CA2, CA4 and neocortex, zero in dentate gyrus, and mild in hippocampal CA3. In contrast, 24 hr after 3-NPA treatment immunoreactivity for bcl-2 protein was strongly upregulated in these brain regions, e.g. in hippocampal CA 1 and CA 3.

In some animals, intensity of bcl-2 immunoreactivity in the respective brain regions was increased already after 3 and 12 hr following 3-NPA injection. After 24 hr all animals presented with significant upregulation of bcl-2 protein in CA 1 (5 out of 5 animals, $p = 0.003$), CA 3 (5/5, $p = 0.003$), CA 4 (4/5, $p = 0.025$) of hippocampus, as well as neocortex (5/5, $p = 0.004$). Neurons in CA 2 and dentate gyrus showed no significant difference in immunoreactivity compared to controls. There was no evidence for neuronal cell damage in any brain region after 3-NPA or vehicle treatment.

Discussion

We observed a time dependent increase in neuronal bcl-2 protein immunoreactivity, induced by a single 3-NPA treatment in brain areas vulnerable to ischemic damage. The apparent increase of bcl-2 protein expression parallels earlier observations of an increased tolerance against global brain ischemia one day after 3-NPA injection ('chemical preconditioning') [17, 21]. This suggests a possible role of bcl-2-protein in chemical induction of tolerance against ischemia in rats. Protein expression [3] is in a good temporal relationship with the upregulation of bcl-2 mRNA in rats treated with 3-NPA accordingly [4].

Bcl-2 protein, an oncoprotein, is present on the cytosolic membrane of mitochondria, on the nuclear envelope, and the endoplasmic reticulum, and appears to sense the actual state of these cell structures. In concert with other pro-survival proteins, bcl-2 is considered a key regulator of apoptosis [for review: 1]. Bcl-2 may act as a death inhibitor through several different mechanisms.

Firstly, bcl-2 protein is thought to inhibit the activation process of cell death promoting proteins (e.g. caspases 1, 4 and 10) via Apaf-1 regulation [1]. However, recent work is challenging this model [16].

Secondly, bcl-2 appears to control the mitochondrial membranes via the mitochondrial permeability transition pore (PT) or mitochondrial megachannel [25]. These multiprotein complexes are formed at the contact site between the mitochondrial inner and outer membranes and regulate the transmembrane proton gradient, pH and calcium levels, as well as the non-selective flux of ions and various proteins between mitochondria and the cytosol. Bcl-2 appears to inhibit PT pore opening, thereby antagonizing the activity of pro-apoptotic proteins (e.g. bax) which facilitate opening or are even constituents of the PT pore [25].

Thirdly, bcl-2 may exert its anti-apoptotic activity through regulation of reactive oxygen species (ROS), thereby reducing the deleterious effects on various cell compartments at times of oxidative stress, e.g. ischemia/reperfusion. Bcl-2 was found to inhibit ROS generation [7, 11], increases levels of ROS scavenger, e.g. superoxide dismutase or gluthatione [8, 15], or may itself act as a free radical scavenger [9].

The cell-survival activities of bcl-2 family proteins are antagonized by pro-apoptotic molecules (e.g. bax) via heterodimerisation with one another. Thus, whether or not certain biological events subsequently lead to an initiation of the cell death program seems to be in part dependent on the intracellular balance between pro-survival, e.g. bcl-2, and pro-apoptotic, e.g. bax, protein levels. However, there are some death signals which apparently bypass bcl-2 control [2].

For this model of chemical preconditioning using a single dose of 3-NPA, we suggest that the increase in bcl-2-protein expression may be initiated by an increase of ROS levels after 3-NPA administration [23]. After a subsequent ischemia/reperfusion more bcl-2 protein is available (i) to control the postischemic ROS burst and/or (ii) to protect mitochondrial membranes from loosing their barrier function, and to prevent the release of intermembrane proteins, e.g. cytochrome c, and/or (iii) to inhibit the activation of cell death-promoting mechanisms via, e.g. caspases.

At this point we would like to emphasize that our current preconditioning technique via a cell toxin (3-NPA) can only serve as a tool to demonstrate that chemical tolerance is feasible, and to understand the underlying mechanisms under experimental conditions. 3-NPA is certainly not suitable for clinical use. However, identifying the important intracellular steps necessary for the induction of tolerance to ischemia will enable us to find or design other, safer substances for 'chemical preconditioning' in patients.

Which patients may benefit from a viable concept of chemical induction of cerebral ischemic tolerance? Several interventions on brain vessels (e.g. aneurysm surgery) or on large arteries (ascending aorta, pulmonary arteries) involve temporary blood flow interruption (e.g. clipping) or even complete circulatory arrest for a certain period. Other surgical procedures are associated with cerebral ischemia and bear the risk of a post-operative neurological deficit, e.g. heart surgery, or carotid endarterectomy. Thus, induction of ischemic tolerance by means of a chemical substance given e.g. one day before surgery, could improve post-operative outcome and the long-term quality of life in all patients were an interruption of blood flow to the brain can be anticipated.

Conclusions

In summary, the results suggest an important role for bcl-2 protein in chemically induced tolerance. Increased expression of bcl-2 24 hr after 3-NPA application may represent a central mechanism for cell protection during subsequent global cerebral ischemia/reperfusion. Many issues, especially the entire cascade triggered by 3-NPA or other, possibly less toxic substances, which can trigger cerebral ischemic tolerance need to be further elucidated before the principle can find its way into everyday clinical practice.

References

1. Adams JM, Cory S (1998) The bcl-2 protein family: Arbiters of cell survival. Science 281: 1322–1326
2. Ashkenazi A, Dixit VM (1998) Death receptors: signaling and modulation. Science 281: 1305–1308
3. Brambrink A, Noga H, Astheimer A, Götz B, Körner I, Heimann A, Kempski O (2001) Bcl-2 protein is upregulated after chemical preconditioning using 3-NPA. In: Maturation phenomenon in cerebral ischemia IV, Springer, Berlin Heidelberg New York Tokyo pp 135–140
4. Brambrink A, Schneider A, Noga H, Astheimer A, Götz B, Körner I, Heimann A, Bach A, Kempski O (2000) Tolerance-inducing dose of 3-nitropropionic acid modulates bcl-2 and bax balance in the rat brain: a potential mechanism of chemical preconditioning. J Cereb Blood Flow Metab 20: 1425–1436
5. Chen J, Graham SH, Nakayama M, Zhu RL, Jin K, Stetler RA, Simon RP (1997) Apoptosis repressor genes bcl-2 and bcl-x-long are expressed in the rat brain following global ischemia. J Cereb Blood Flow Metab 17: 2–10
6. Christensen T, Bruhn T, Balchen T, Diemer NH (1994) Evidence for formation of hydroxyl radicals during reperfusion after global cerebral ischemia in rats using salicylate trapping and microdialysis. Neurobiol Dis 1: 131–138
7. Ellerby HM, Martin SJ, Ellerby LM, Naiem SS, Rabizadeh S, Salvesen GS, Casiano CA, Cashman NR, Green DR, Bredesen DE (1997) Establishment of a cell-free system of neuronal apoptosis: comparison of premitochondrial, mitochondrial, and postmitochondrial phases. J Neurosci 17: 6165–6178
8. Ellerby LM, Ellerby HM, Park SM, Holleran AL, Murphy AN, Fiskum G, Kane DJ, Testa MP, Kayalar C, Bredesen DE (1996) Shift of the cellular oxidation-reduction potential in neural cells expressing Bcl-2. J Neurochem 67: 1259–1267
9. Hockenbery DM, Oltvai ZN, Yin XM, Milliman CL, Korsmeyer SJ (1993) Bcl-2 functions in an antioxidant pathway to prevent apoptosis. Cell 75: 241–251
10. Hu S, Sheng WS, Peterson PK, Chao CC (1995) Cytokine modulation of murine microglia cell superoxide production. Glia 13: 45–50
11. Kane DJ, Sarafian TA, Anton R, Hahn H, Gralla EB, Valentine JS, Örd T, Bredesen DE (1993) Bcl-2 Inhibition of neural death: decreased generation of reactive oxygen species. Science 262: 1274–1277
12. Kato H, Kogure K, Araki T, Liu X-H, Kato K, Itoyama Y (1995) Immunohistochemical localization of superoxide dismutase in the hippocampus following ischemia in a gerbil model of ischemic tolerance. J Cereb Blood Flow Metab 15: 60–70
13. Kinouchi H, Epstein CJ, Mizui T, Carlson E, Chen SF, Chan PH (1991) Attenuation of focal cerebral ischemic injury in transgenic mice overexpressing CuZn superoxide dismutase. Proc Natl Acad Sci USA 88: 11158–11162
14. Lauritzen M, Hansen AJ, Kronborg D, Wieloch T (1990) Cortical spreading depression is associated with arachidonic acid accumulation and preservation of energy charge. J Cereb Blood Flow Metab 10: 115–122
15. Meredith MJ, Cusick CL, Soltaniassab S, Sekhar KS, Lu S, Freemann ML (1998) Expression of bcl-2 increase intracellular glutathione by inhibiting methionine-dependent GSH efflux. Biochem Biophys Res Com 248: 458–463
16. Moriishi K, Huang DS, Cory S, Adams JM (1999) Bcl-2 famili members do not inhibit apoptosis by binding the caspase activator Apaf-1. Proc Natl Acad Sci USA 96: 9683–9688
17. Nakase H, Heimann A, Uranishi R, Riepe MW, Kempski O (2000) Early-onset tolerance to rat global cerebral ischemia induced by a mitochondrial inhibitor. Neurosci Letters 290: 105–108
18. Riepe MW, Esclaire F, Kasischke K, Schreiber S, Nakase H, Kempski O, Ludolph AC, Dirnagl U, Hugon J (1997) Increased hypoxic tolerance by chemical inhibition of oxydative phosphorylation: chemical preconditioning. J Cereb Blood Flow Metab 17: 257–264
19. Siesjö BK, Agardh CD, Bengtsson F (1989) Free radicals and brain damage. Cerebrovasc Brain Metab Rev 1: 165–211
20. Simon RP, Chen J (1996) Apoptosis receptor gene bcl-2; potential role in ischemia tolerance. In: Krieglstein J, Oberpichler-

Schwenk H (eds) Pharmacology of cerebral ischemia 1996. Medpharm Scientific Publisher, Stuttgart, pp 25–31
21. Sugino T, Nozaki K, Tagagi Y, Hashimoto N (1999) 3-Nitropropionic acid induces ischemic tolerance in gerbil hippocampus in vivo. Neurosc Lett 259: 9–12
22. Toyoda T, Kassell NF, Lee KS (1997) Induction of ischemic tolerance and antioxidant activity by brief focal ischemia. Neuroreport 8: 847–851
23. Wiegand F, Lindauer U, Busch C, Liao W, Megow D, Dirnagl U (1997) Tolerance to focal ischemia induced by 3-Nitropropionic acid (3-NPA) is mediated by formation of reactive oxygen species (ROS). Soc Neurosci Abstr 23: 2183
24. Xu DG, Crocker SJ, Doucet JP, St.-Jean M, Tamai K, Hakim AM, Ikeda JE, Liston P, Thompson CS, Kornelik RG, MacKenzie A, Robertson GS (1997) Elevation of neuronal expression of NAIP reduces ischemic damage in the rat hippocampus. Nat Med 3: 997–1004
25. Zamzami N, Brenner C, Marzo I, Susin SA, Kroemer G (1998) Subcellular and submitochondrial mode of bcl-2-like oncoproteins. Oncogene 16: 2265–2282

Correspondence: Prof. Dr. med. O. Kempski, Institut of Neurosurgical Pathophysiology, Johannes Gutenberg-University, D-55131 Mainz, Germany. e-mail: kempski@nc-patho.klinik.uni-mainz.de

Traumatic brain and spinal cord injury – the experimental approach

Acta Neurochir (2004) [Suppl] 89: 69–74

Printed in Austria

The role of inflammatory processes in the pathophysiology and treatment of brain and spinal cord trauma

W. D. Dietrich, K. Chatzipanteli, E. Vitarbo, K. Wada, and **K. Kinoshita**

Department of Neurological Surgery, Neurotrauma Research Center, Miami Project to Cure Paralysis, University of Miami School of Medicine, Miami, FL USA

Summary

Traumatic injury to the brain and spinal cord results in an early inflammatory response that is initiated by the release of pro-inflammatory cytokines followed by the infiltration and accumulation of polymorphonuclear leukocytes (PMNLs). The role of the inflammatory cascade on traumatic outcome remains controversial. Pleiotropic cytokines appear to function both protectively and destructively. The induction of cytokines can lead to the expression of the inducible form of nitric oxide synthase (iNOS), which in turn provokes the release of excessive amounts of nitric oxide (NO) that may participate in the pathogenesis of tissue injury. Hypothermia has been reported by various groups to be neuroprotective in brain and spinal cord trauma. We studied the effect of therapeutic hypothermia on cerebral IL-1β concentrations, PMNL accumulation and iNOS activity after traumatic brain injury (TBI) and spinal cord injury (SCI). Based on current data therapeutic hypothermia may protect in models of traumatic injury by modulating deleterious inflammatory processes.

Keywords: Traumatic brain injury (TBI); Spinal cord injury (SCI); Interleukin-1 beta (IL-1β); hypothermia.

Introduction

Traumatic brain (TBI) and spinal cord injury (SCI) initiates a cascade of acute and more chronic inflammatory processes that influence outcome. While more acute inflammatory processes are felt to worsen outcome, recent data indicate that more delayed inflammatory processes may participate in reparative processes [41, 44, 46, 47]. Thus, there is a continued need to clarify what specific inflammatory events should be targeted for acute neuroprotective strategies without affecting more delayed processes that may promote improvement. Much work has been accomplished in various models of brain and spinal cord trauma that have helped clarify the cellular and molecular events that lead to the recruitment of inflammatory cells [18, 23, 42, 51, 52]. Ongoing research in our laboratory is concentrated on therapeutic strategies that target acute and subacute inflammatory processes with the goal of improving histopathological and functional outcome in established injury models. This chapter reports recent data on TBI and SCI and summarizes treatment studies including therapeutic hypothermia that appear to target multiple inflammatory cellular events.

Pro-inflammatory cytokine IL-1β

Traumatic brain injury is associated with the production and release of pro-inflammatory cytokines including tumor necrotic factor-alpha (TNF-α), Interleukin-1beta (IL-1β) and Interleukin-6 (IL-6) [47, 50]. IL-1β is the key mediator of the acute inflammatory response following cerebral ischemia and brain trauma. Cytokines mediate multiple cellular functions ranging from neuroprotective to neurotoxic effects. Various in vivo studies have strongly implicated IL-1β as a significant pro-inflammatory mediator of secondary injury [63]. Increased protein levels of IL-1β have been demonstrated in brain tissue and blood from patients with brain trauma, stroke and other neurological diseases [15, 18]. This cytokine is also expressed in response to other stimuli including infection or seizures [43]. IL-1β is a potent enhancer of inflammatory reactions through the release of other inflammatory mediators such as prostaglandin, collagenase and phospholipase A_2 [42]. This cytokine has been implicated in such diverse processes as apoptotic cell death [30], leukocyte-endothelial adhesion [5], blood-

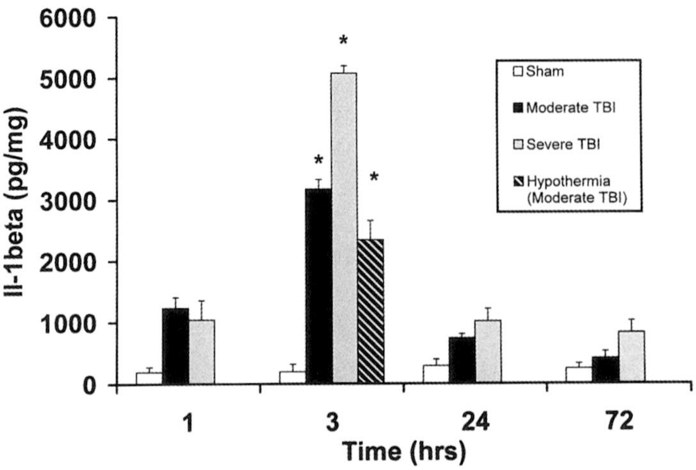

Fig. 1. Time course of IL-1β concentration as measured by ELISA in cytosolic extracts of injured cerebral cortex following moderate and severe TBI. IL-1β also measured 3 hours after post-traumatic hypothermia (33 °C). Bar graphs illustrate means ± SEM (n = 4 per group) (*$p < 0.05$ indicate statistical difference compared with sham-operated rats)

brain barrier disruption [39], edema formation [30, 63], astrogliosis [28], neurovascularization [28] and the synthesis of neurotrophic factors [17]. Although cytokine actions in the brain have most often been considered to participate in damaging processes, these inflammatory mediators also act as neuromodulators in the intact brain [42, 55]. In this regard, IL-1β and its mRNA are present in the normal rat brain [1, 24, 65]. Finally, inflammation has also been suggested to contribute to brain healing mainly through processes associated with the removal of damaged tissue [29, 42].

In experimental studies, the inhibition of IL-1β has been reported to reduce lesion size after brain trauma [54] and decrease early edema formation [64]. For example, early treatment with recombinant human interleukin-1β receptor antagonist (rh IL-1ra) in the rat brain reduces lesion volume [54]. Although these observations implicate IL-1β in secondary injury cascade, other studies have shown lack of protection with IL-1β antagonists following brain trauma [33]. Novel therapeutic approaches that block the cytotoxic actions of IL-1β require additional investigation in studies where chronic histopathological and behavioral studies are used as endpoints.

Previous studies from our laboratory have documented the beneficial effects of posttraumatic hypothermia on histopathological and functional outcome [9, 19]. We recently investigated the temporal and regional profiles of IL-1β in brain tissue as well as changes in the concentration of IL-1β under posttraumatic hypothermic conditions. Male Sprague-Dawley rats underwent moderate (1.8–2.2 atm) or severe (2.4–2.7 atm) parasagittal fluid percussion brain injury [21]. In hypothermic animals, systemic temperature was reduced to 33 °C for 3 hours beginning 15 minutes after trauma. IL-1β levels of the lesion were quantified using an ELISA IL-1β assay after a three-hour period of normothermia or hypothermia. Results indicate that severe and moderate TBI induce increasing levels of IL-1β within the injured brain at all time points tested, with the most robust increase observed at 3 hrs (Fig. 1). Hypothermia (33 °C) attenuated IL-1β levels in the injured right cortex as compared to the normothermic group after moderate TBI. However, the concentration of IL-1β was still elevated compared to sham-operated controls. These results indicate that injury severity is an important factor for the production of pro-inflammatory cytokines and that early post-traumatic hypothermia may reduce systemic inflammation through modulating IL-1β production.

Neutrophil accumulation after traumatic brain and spinal cord injury

Polymorphonuclear leukocyte (PMNL) accumulation after brain and spinal cord injury has been implicated in the pathogenesis of neuronal injury [45]. Although the acute accumulation of neutrophils observed after F-P brain injury may represent hemorrhage associated with primary vascular injury [14, 20, 45, 53], neutrophil accumulation remains elevated for several days as a consequence of active recruitment mechanisms [10, 59]. Neutrophils may contribute to neuronal damage by the release of oxygen radical metabolites, hydrolytic enzymes and cytokines [45, 52]. Early neutrophil accumulation after TBI could contribute to tissue injury by releasing pro-inflammatory cytokines. Anti-inflammatory strategies targeting neu-

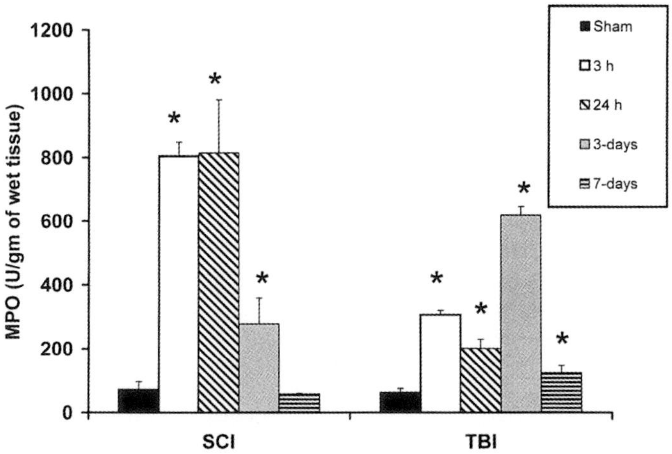

Fig. 2. Time course of myeloperoxidase (MPO) activity in the injured T10 spinal cord region and cerebral cortex after SCI or TBI, respectively. Within the injured T10 region, a significant increase in MPO activity was observed at 3, 24 hrs or 3-days after contusion, with peak values observed at 3 and 24 hrs. In the traumatized cerebral cortex, a significant increase of MPO activity was observed at 3 and 24 hr, and 3 and 7 days, with peak values at 3 days (n = 4 per group) (significantly different from sham operated rats $*p < 0.05$)

trophil accumulation may therefore be an important therapeutic strategy to reduce neural damage following TBI.

Recently, we have investigated the regional and temporal profile of PMNL accumulation in rat models of TBI and SCI. Following moderate parasagittal F-P brain injury, neutrophil accumulation as determined by the regional enzymatic activity of myeloperoxidase (MPO) significantly increased at 3, 24 hrs, 3 and 7-days (Fig. 2) [11]. MPO values peaked at the 3-day period. Following contusion injury of the T10 thoracic spinal cord using the New York University (NYU) impactor, massive neutrophil accumulation was documented at 3, 24 and 72 hours after injury [13], with peak values observed at 24 hrs. Interestingly, elevated levels of MPO activity were more acute and severe after spinal cord injury versus traumatic brain injury. In both TBI and SCI experiments, post-traumatic hypothermia (30 °C and 32 °C, respectively) significantly decreased MPO activity as compared to normothermic animals [11, 13]. Thus, post-traumatic hypothermia may also be neuroprotective in models of brain and spinal cord injury by reducing acute PMNL accumulation.

iNOS activity after TBI and SCI

Nitric oxide (NO) has been reported to play an important role in the pathophysiology of TBI and cerebral ischemia [40, 56]. It is known that under physiological conditions, the inducible form of NOS (iNOS) is absent from mammalian cells. However, in pathological conditions, iNOS is activated at the transcriptional level as a result of proinflammatory stimuli, including bacterial lipopolysaccharide or proinflammatory cytokines [49]. The combination of multiple cytokines has also been reported to result in NO production by iNOS [38]. As previously discussed, several cytokines are expressed in the injured brain and within the cerebrospinal fluid after TBI [15, 38, 62]. Astrocytes [25, 26, 58], and macrophages/microglia [6, 27, 34] can express iNOS in vitro and mediate neuronal cell death after injury. The expression of iNOS has also been observed in other cell types including endothelial cells, vascular smooth muscle cells and oligodendroglia following various pathophysiological conditions [8, 35]. In in vivo models, these cells can become activated and the activation is most prominent after one day [53].

Previous studies have demonstrated that once iNOS is expressed, it produces NO continuously at considerably increased levels compared with basal NO production [52, 57]. The potential mechanisms of the sustained production of NO in the injured brain have been discussed [16, 31, 37, 57, 60]. NO-induced cytotoxicity may involve the inhibition of cellular energy production by the inhibition of the glycolytic enzyme glyceraldehyde-3-phosphate dehydrogenase (GAPDH) [22] and the mitochondrial enzymes *cis*-aconitase and complexes I and II. In addition, NO also produces DNA damage, inhibits DNA replication by inhibiting ribonucleotide reductase, and triggers apoptosis [7]. DNA damage activates poly adenosine 5'diphosphoribose synthetase (PARS), an enzyme that may lead to neurotoxicity by the depletion of essential substrates and ATP [36, 66]. In biological systems, NO can also cause toxicity, mainly through the diffusion-limited reaction of NO with superoxide anion (O_2^-)

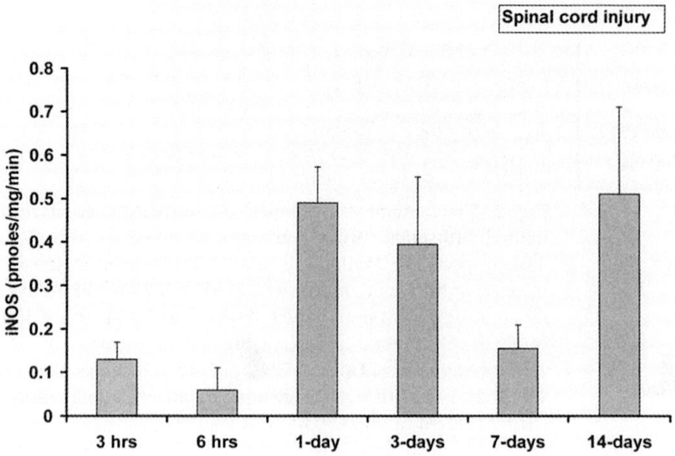

Fig. 3. Time course of iNOS activity in the injured spinal cord segment (T10), following moderate spinal cord injury *(SCI)*. Significantly elevated iNOS activity was detected at 3, 6, 24 hrs and 7 and 14-days after SCI. The largest increase was seen at 24 hr after SCI, (n = 4 per group)

to generate peroxynitrite (ONOO-) [2, 3, 61] and promote oxidative damage by perturbing iron metabolism.

Recently, we have determined the time course of iNOS enzymatic activity after TBI and SCI [11, 57]. Following moderate F-P injury, iNOS activity is significantly increased in the injured cortical area at 3 days and peaks at 7 days posttrauma. In contrast, following moderate SCI, iNOS activity is significantly increased at the injury site at 3, 6 and 24 hours, 3, 7 and 14-days after injury (Fig. 3). Interestingly, double label immunocytochemical staining of iNOS demonstrated that a large number of immunopositive cells were PMNLs. Thus, the early accumulation of PMNLs after brain and spinal cord injury appear to be a potential source of NO induced cytotoxic products. Finally, posttraumatic hypothermia (30 °C/3 hrs) significantly decreased the elevation of iNOS activity at 7 days after TBI. Taken together, these data indicate that posttraumatic hypothermia may be neuroprotective by decreasing iNOS activity.

Interleukin-10 after TBI and SCI

In addition to posttraumatic hypothermia, specific pharmacological strategies have been used to target acute inflammatory processes [17, 19, 46, 50, 54, 64]. For example, recent data indicate that interleukin-10 (IL-10) a potent anti-inflammatory cytokine is neuroprotective in models of brain and spinal cord injury [4, 32, 48]. Most recently, acute administration IL-10 has been shown to reduce TNF-α synthesis and to improve both histopathological and behavioral outcome in a model of SCI [4]. Interestingly, while acute treatment of IL-10 was neuroprotective, acute and more chronic treatment did not lead to a similar improvement in outcome. These data emphasize the potential of inflammatory processes following CNS injury to result in both detrimental as well as beneficial consequences in terms of recovery of function [3]. Additional investigations are therefore necessary to clarify the therapeutic windows for strategies that target inflammation after injury and to clarify detrimental as well as beneficial inflammatory events. Combination therapies, possibly including hypothermia plus pharmacological agents that target specific inflammatory processes, may be beneficial in treating patients with brain and spinal cord injury.

Acknowledgments

These investigations were supported by 5P50 NS 30291-10 and 1PO1 NS38665-01A2 from the National Institutes of Health. The authors thank Susan Kraydieh and Dr. Alex Marcillo for expert technical support and Charlaine Rowlette for editorial assistance and manuscript preparation.

References

1. Bandtlow CE, Meyer M, Lindholm D, Spranger M, Heumann R, Thoenen H (1990) Regional and cellular codistribution of interleukin 1 beta and nerve growth factor mRNA in the adult rat brain: possible relationship to the regulation of nerve growth factor synthesis. J Cell Biol 111(4): 1701–1711
2. Beckman JS, Beckman TW, Chen J, Marshal PA, Freeman BA (1990) Apparent hydroxyl radical production by peroxynitrite:

implications for endothelial injury from nitric oxide and superoxide. Proc Natl Acad Sci USA 87: 1620–1624
3. Beckman JS, Koppenol WH (1996) Nitric oxide, superoxide, and peroxynitrite: the good, the bad, and the ugly. Cell Physiol 40: C1424–C1437
4. Bethea JR, Nagashima H, Acosta MC, Briceno C, Marcillo AE, Loor K, Green J, Dietrich DW (1999) Systemically administered interleukin-10 reduces tumor necrosis factor-alpha production following traumatic spinal cord injury in rats. J Neurotrauma 16: 851–861
5. Bevilacqua MP, Pober JS, Wheeler ME, Cotran RS, Gimbrone MA (1985) Interleukin 1 acts on cultured human vascular endothelium to increase the adhesion of polymorphonuclear leukocytes, monocytes, and related leukocyte cell lines. J Clin Invest 76: 2003–2011
6. Boje KM, Arora PK (1992) Microglial-produced nitric oxide and reactive oxides mediate neuronal cell death. Brain Res 587: 250–256
7. Bonfoco E, Krainc D, Ankarcrona M, Nicotera P, Lipton SA (1995) Apoptosis and necrosis: two distinct events induced, respectively, by mild and intense insults with N-methyl-D-aspartate or nitric oxide/superoxide in cortical cell cultures. Proc Natl Acad Sci USA 92: 7162–7166
8. Bonmann E, Suschek C, Spranger M, Kolb-Bachofen V (1997) The dominant role of exogenous interleukin-1 beta on expression and activity of inducible nitric oxide synthase in rat microvascular brain endothelial cells. Neurosci Lett 230: 109–112
9. Bramlett HM, Green EJ, Dietrich WD, Busto R, Globus MY-T, Ginsgerg MD (1995) Posttraumatic brain hypothermia provides protection from sensorimotor and cognitive deficits. J Neurotrauma 12: 289–298
10. Carlos TM, Clark RS, Franicola-Higgins D, Schiding JK, Kochanek PM (1997) Expression of endothelial adhesion molecules and recruitment of neutrophils after traumatic brain injury in rats. J Leukoc Biol 61: 279–285
11. Chatzipanteli K, Alonso OF, Kraydieh S, Dietrich WD (2000) Importance of posttraumatic hypothermia and hyperthermia on the inflammatory response after fluid percussion brain injury: biochemical and immunocytochemical studies. J Cereb Blood Flow Metab 20: 531–542
12. Chatzipanteli K, Garcia R, Marcillo AE, Kraydieh S, Dietrich WD (2001) Temporal and regional distribution of constitutive and inducible nitric oxide synthases following spinal cord injury (submitted)
13. Chatzipanteli K, Yanagawa Y, Marcillo AE, Kraydieh S, Yezierski RP, Dietrich WD (2000) Posttraumatic hypothermia reduces polymorphonuclear leukocyte accumulation following spinal cord injury in rats. J Neurotrauma 17: 321–332
14. Cortez SC, McIntosh TK, Noble LJ (1989) Experimental fluid percussion brain injury: vascular disruption and neuronal and glial alterations. Brain Res 482(2): 271–282
15. Csuka E, Morganti-Kossman MC, Lenzlinger PM, Joller H, Trentz O, Kossmann T (1999) IL-10 levels in cerebrospinal fluid and serum of patients with severe traumatic brain injury: relationship to IL-6, TNF-alpha, TGF-beta1 and blood-brain barrier function. J Neuroimmunol 101: 211–221
16. Dawson VL, Dawson TM, Bartley DA, Uhl GR, Snyder SH (1993) Mechanisms of nitric oxide-mediated neurotoxicity in primary brain cultures. J Neurosci 13: 2651–2661
17. DeKosky ST, Styren SD, O'Malley ME, Goss JR, Kochanek P, Marion D, Evans CH, Robbins PD (1996) Interleukin-1 receptor antagonist suppresses neurotrophin response in injured rat brain. Ann Neurol 39: 123–127
18. del Zoppo G, Ginis I, Hallenbeck JM, Iadecola C, Wang X, Feuerstein GZ (2000) Inflammation and stroke: putative role for cytokines, adhesion molecules and iNOS in brain response to ischemia. Brain Pathol 10: 95–112
19. Dietrich DW, Busto R, Bethea JR (1999) Post-ischemic hypothermia and IL-10 treatment provide long-term neuroprotection of CA1 hippocampus following transient global ischemia in rats. Exp. Neurology 158: 444–450
20. Dietrich WD, Alonso O, Busto R, Globus MY, Ginsberg MD (1994) Post-traumatic brain hypothermia reduces histopathological damage following concussive brain injury in the rat. Acta Neuropathol (Berl) 87: 250–258
21. Dietrich WD, Alonso O, Halley M (1994) Early microvascular and neuronal consequences of traumatic brain injury: a light and electron microscopic study in rats. J Neurotrauma 11: 289–301
22. Dimmeler S, Lottspeich F, Brune B (1992) Nitric oxide causes ADP-ribosylation and inhibition of glyceraldehyde-3-phosphate dehydrogenase. J Biol Chem 267: 16771–16774
23. Dirnagl U, Iadecola C, Moskowitz MA (1999) Pathobiology of ischaemic stroke: an integrated view. Trends Neurosci 22: 391–397
24. Freidlander RM, Gagliardini V, Rotello RJ, and Yuan J (1996) Functional role of interleukin 1 beta in IL-1 beta-converting enzyme-mediated apoptosis. J Exp Med 184: 717–724
25. Galea E, Feinstein DL, Reis D (1992) Induction of calcium-independent nitric oxide synthase activity in primary rat glial cultures. Proc Natl Acad Sci USA 89: 10945–10949
26. Galea E, Reis DJ, Feinstein DL (1994) Cloning and expression of inducible nitric oxide syntahase from rat astrocytes. J Neurosci Res 37: 406–414
27. Garthwaite J (1991) Glutamate, nitric oxide and cell-cell signalling in the nervous system. Trends Neurosci 14: 60–67
28. Giulian D, Woodward J, Young DG, Krebs JF, Lachman LB (1988) Interleukin-1 injected into mammalian brain stimulates astrogliosis and neovascularization. J Neurosci 8: 2485–2490
29. Hays SJ (1998) Therapeutic approaches to the treatment of neuroinflammatory diseases. Curr Pharm Des 4: 335–348
30. Holmin S, Mathiesen T (2000) Intracerebral administration of interleukin-1beta and induction of inflammation, apoptosis, and vasogenic edema. J Neurosurg 92: 108–120
31. Iadecola C (1997) Bright and dark sides of nitric oxide in ischemic brain injury. Trends Neurosci 20: 132–139
32. Knoblach SM, Faden AI (1998) Interleukin-10 improves outcome and alters proinflammtory cytokine expression after experimental traumatic brain injury. Exp Neurol 153: 143–151
33. Knoblach SM, Faden AI (2000) Cortical interleukin-1β elevation after traumatic brain injury in the rat: no effect of two selective antagonists on motor recovery Neuroscience Letters 289: 5–8
34. Kong LY, McMillian MK, Maronpot R, Hong JS (1996) Protein tyrosine kinase inhibitors suppress the production of nitric oxide in mixed glia, microglia-enriched or astrocyte-enriched cultures. Brain Res 729: 102–109
35. Merrill JE, Murphy SP, Mitrovic B, Mackenzie-Graham A, Dopp JC, Ding M, Griscavage J, Ignarro LJ, Lowenstein CJ (1997) Inducible nitric oxide synthase and nitric oxide production by oligodendrocytes. J Neurosci Res 48: 372–384
36. Nathan C, Xie QW (1994) Regulation of biosynthesis of nitric oxide. J Biol Chem 269: 13725–13728
37. Nathan C (1992) Nitric oxide as a secretory product of mammalian cells. FASEB J 6: 3051–3064
38. Ott L, McClain CJ, Gillespie M, Young B (1994) Cytokines and metabolic dysfunction after severe head injury. J Neurotrauma 11: 447–472

39. Quagliarello VJ, Wispelwey B, Long WJ, Scheld WM (1991) Recombinant human interleukin-1 induces meningitis and blood-brain barrier injury in the rat. Characterization and comparison with tumor necrosis factor. J Clin Invest 87: 1360–1366
40. Rao AM, Dogan A, Hatcher JF, Dempsey RJ (1998) Fluorometric assay of nitrite and nitrate in brain tissue after traumatic brain injury and cerebral ischemia. Brain Res 793: 265–270
41. Rapalino O, Lazarov-Spiegler O, Agranov E, Velan GJ, Yoles E, Fraidakis M, Solomon A, Gepstein R, Katz A, Belkin M, Hadani, Swartz M (1998) Implantation of stimulated homologous macrophages results in partial recovery of paraplegic rats. Nature Medicine 4: 814–821
42. Rothwell NJ (1999) Annual review prize lecture cytokines – killers in the brain? J Physiol 3: 514–517
43. Rothwell NJ, Loddick SA, Stroemer P (1997) Interleukins and cerebral ischaemia. Int Rev Neurobiol 40: 281–298
44. Scherbel U, Raghupathi R, Nakamura M, Saatman KE, Trojanowski JQ, Neugebauer E, Marino MW, McIntosh TK (1999) Differential acute and chronic responses of tumor necrosis factor-deficient mice to experimental brain injury. Proc Natl Acad Sci USA 96: 8721–8726
45. Schoettle RJ, Kochanek PM, Magargee MJ, Uhl MW, Nemoto EM (1990) Early polymorphonuclear leukocyte accumulation correlates with the development of posttraumatic cerebral edema in rats. J Neurotrauma 7: 207–217
46. Shohami E, Bass R, Wallach D, Yamin A, Gallily R (1996) Inhibition of tumor necrosis factor alpha (TNF-α) activity in rat brain is associated with cerebroprotection after closed head injury. J Cereb Blood Flow Metab 16: 378–384
47. Shohami E, Ginis I, Hallenbeck JM (1999) Dual role of tumor necrosis factor alpha in brain injury. Cytokine and Growth Factors Reviews 10: 119–130
48. Spera PA, Ellison JA, Feuerstein GZ, Barone FC (1998) IL-10 reduces brain injury following focal stroke. Neurosci Letters 251: 189–192
49. Szabo C, Thiemermann C (1995) Regulation of the expression of the inducible isoform of nitric oxide synthase. Advance Pharmacol 34: 113–153
50. Taupin V, Toulmond S, Serrano A, Benavides J, Zavala F (1993) Increases in IL-6, IL-1 and TNF levels in rat brain following traumatic lesion. Influence of pre- and post-traumatic treatment with Ro5 4864, a peripheral–type (p site) benzodiazepine ligand. J Neuroimmunology 42: 177–185
51. Tomita M, Fukuuchi Y (1996) Leukocytes, macrophages and secondary brain injury following cerebral ischemia. Acta Neurochir Suppl (Wien) 66: 32–39
52. Tonnesen MG, Worthen GS, Johnston RG (1988) Neutrophil emigration, activation, and tissue damage. In: Clark RAF, Hesen PM (eds) The molecular and Cellular Biology of Wound Repair Plenum, New York, pp. 149–184
53. Toulmond S, Duval D, Serrano A, Scatton B, Benavides J (1993) Biochemical and histological alterations induced by fluid percussion brain injury in the rat. Brain Res 620: 24–31
54. Toulmond S, Rothwell NJ (1995) Interleukin-1 receptor antagonist inhibits neuronal damage caused by fluid percussion injury in the rat. Brain Res 671: 261–266
55. Vitkovic L, Bockaert J, Cjacque C (2000) Inflammatory cytokines. J Neurochemistry 74: 457–471
56. Wada J, Chatzipanteli K, Busto R, Dietrich WD (1998) Role of NO in traumatic brain injury in the rat. J Neurosurgery 89: 807–818
57. Wada K, Chatzipanteli K, Kraydieh S, Busto S, Dietrich WD (1998) Inducible nitric oxide synthase expression after traumatic brain injury and neuroprotection with aminoguanidine treatment in rats. Neurosurgery 43: 1427–1436
58. Wallace MN, Bisland S (1994) NADPH-diaphorase activity in activated astrocytes represents inducible nitric oxide synthase. Neuroscience 59: 905–919
59. Whalen MJ, Carlos TM, Kochanek PM, Clark RS, Heineman S, Schiding JK, Franicola D, Memarzadeh F, Lo W, Marion DW, DeKosky ST (1999) Neutrophils do not mediate blood-brain barrier permeability early after controlled cortical impact in rats. J Neurotrauma 16(7): 583–594
60. Xia QW, Nathan C (1994) The high-output nitric oxide pathway: role and regulation. J Leukoc Biol 56: 576–582
61. Xia Y, Dawson VL, Dawson TM, Snyder SH, Zweier JL (1996) Nitric oxide synthase generates superoxide and nitric oxide in arginine-depleted cells leading to peroxynitrite-mediated cellular injury. Proc Natl Acad Sci USA 93: 6770–6774
62. Yakovlev A, Faden AI (1994) Expression of immediate-early response genes, cytokine and ICAM-1 genes in rat hippocampus following traumatic brain injury. Soc Neurosci Abstr 20: 423
63. Yamasaki Y, Matsuura N, Shozuhara H, Onodera H, Itoyama Y, Kogure K (1995) Interleukin-1 as a pathogenetic mediator of ischemic brain damage in rats. Stroke 26: 676–681
64. Yamasaki Y, Shozuhara H, Onodera H, Kogure K (1994) Blocking of interleukin-1 activity is a beneficial approach to ischemia brain edema formation. Acta Neurochir Suppl (Wien) 60: 300–302
65. Yan HQ, Banos MA, Herregodts P, Hooghe R, Hooghe-Peters EL (1992) Expression of interleukin (IL)-1 beta, IL-6 and their respective receptors in the normal rat brain and after injury. Eur J Immunol 22(11): 2963–2971
66. Zhang J, Dawson VL, Dawson TM, Snyder SH (1994) Nitric oxide activation of poly (ADP-ribose) synthetase in neurotoxicity. Science 263: 687–689

Correspondence: W. Dalton Dietrich, Ph.D., Scientific Director (R-48), The Miami Project to Cure Paralysis P.O. Box 016960, Miami FL 33101, USA. e-mail: ddietrich@miami.edu

Acta Neurochir (2004) [Suppl] 89: 75–80

Printed in Austria

L-type calcium channel antagonist nifedipine reduces neurofilament restitution following traumatic optic nerve injury

J. Hanke and **B. A. Sabel**

Institute of Medical Psychology, Otto-von-Guericke University, Magdeburg, Germany

Summary

Background. The aim of the present study was to observe if the use of the L-type calcium channel antagonist nifedipine would offer advantages for the retinal ganglion cells and the restitution of the axonal cytoskeleton after optic nerve crush.

Methods. Retinal ganglion cells were retrogradely labeled with a fluorescent calcium marker. With the in vivo confocal neuroimaging (ICON) method we observed the fluorescent cell metabolism marker Oregon Green BAPTA in the same retinal ganglion cells over 3 weeks after optic nerve crush. 2 µmol nifedipine were injected intraocularly 30 minutes following optic nerve crush.

Findings. Investigation of the optic nerve immunostained for NF-H presented decreased restitution of the neurofilaments in the axonal cytoskeleton after 3 weeks in the optic nerve crush group treated with nifedipine as compared to the optic nerve crush only group.

Interpretation. These results show that a single injection of the calcium L-type antagonist nifedipine shortly after optic nerve injury has long-lasting negative effects on the recovery of the retinal ganglion cells.

Keywords: Retinal ganglion cells; recovery; calcium imaging; in vivo imaging.

Introduction

Abnormal accumulation of intracellular calcium following traumatic brain injury (TBI) is thought to contribute to a cascade of cellular events that lead to pathological conditions. Therefore, the possibility that specific calcium channel antagonists might exert neuroprotective effects in TBI has been of interest because smaller variations of the frequencies and/or the amplitudes of calcium signals are necessary for normal cell functions [2]. Only 30 min after induction of ischemia neurones develop cytoplasmic vacuolation while accumulation of calcium in swollen mitochondria was demonstrated by the use of the cytochemical pyroantimonate technique [9, 31]. In addition to mitochondrial changes in axons there was loss of axonal microtubules and disorganisation of neurofilaments [19, 32].

Initial stages after diffuse axon injury (DAI) include not only changes of the cytoskeleton [12, 22, 23, 27] but also disturbance of the axonal transport [15]. The damage of neurofilament (NF) structure in the cytoskeleton of axons induced by mechanical deformation during trauma is thought to cause regional compaction and/or impaired transport. As a result, accumulation of transport material induces regional axonal swelling [21]. Ionic shifts and secondary activation of proteases lead to degradation of the axonal ultrastructure. In the DAI model of the optic nerve crush (ONC) [5] there is evidence that despite death of about 85% of the retinal ganglion cells (RGCs) [3] recovery of vision occurs after initial blindness [30]. This functional recovery is highly correlated with the morphological appearance of the surviving RGCs [25], the restitution of the cytoskeleton and restoration of the axonal transport [7]. Recovery of physiological function was observed in a relative short period after DAI in both humans [4] and experimental animals [24], which cannot be explained by time consuming regeneration of axons. Therefore, nondisrupted axons play a special role in recovery of function [6, 29], and they may, for example, contribute to recovery of vision in humans as well [11]. For this reason the establishment of prospective manipulations to accelerate functional recovery has to be started shortly after injury.

The intention of the present study was to prevent calcium induced cell death and acceleration of functional recovery after ONC. Therefore, L-type calcium channel antagonist nifedipine that is widely used in patients after TBI was intraocularly injected 30 minutes after ONC. The RGCs were observed with the in vivo confocal neuroimaging (ICON) method [28], which allows repeated visualization of the same cells over time. After 14 and 21 days respectively, the left and right optic nerves were dissected, followed by immunostaining for NF-H and investigation of the axonal skeleton.

Materials and methods

Subjects

Adult male Wistar rats (Harlan Winkelmann GmbH, Borchens, Germany) were used for this study. All experiments were carried out in accordance with the German Law on the Protection of Animals and protocols were approved by legal authorities (Tierversuchsgenehmigung Nr. Psy/G/1/99). The animals were kept under a 12 h light/12 h dark cycle with free access to water and food with lights on at 6.00 a.m.. 15 animals were used (5 rats ONC and nifedipine, 5 rats ONC only, 5 rats sham-operated).

ONC

A bilateral optic nerve crush was carried out as described before [5, 30] under anaesthesia (ketamine 50 mg/kg–rompun 10 mg/kg, i.p., Parke-Davis, Berlin – Bayer, Leverkusen, Germany). In short: The optic nerve was approached from the orbita by a lateral canthotomy under the guidance of a surgical microscope. The optic nerve was exposed by blunt dissection, leaving both retinal blood supply and dura intact. The nerve was crushed with a calibrated forceps at a distance of 3 mm from the eye for a duration of 30 s. After completion of the crush, the canthotomy was sutured and an antibiotic eye ointment was topically applied to prevent inflammation (Aureomycin, Lederle Arzneimittel GmbH, Wolfratshausen, Germany). Surgery for control animals was performed leaving the optic nerve intact.

Injections of the calcium marker

RGCs were labelled retrogradely under anaesthesia (ketamine 50 mg/kg–rompun 10 mg/kg, i.p.). Calcium activity in the RGCs was measured after injection of 2 μl Oregon Green BAPTA-dextran (dilution 1:5 in bidistiled water, Molecular Probes, Leiden, Netherlands) into the right and left superior colliculus before ONC (10 animals, coordinates: anterior-posterior 6.5 mm, lateral 1.4 mm and −1.4 mm, 3.0–3.5 mm below dura).

To study the effect of the L-type calcium channel antagonist nifedipine after ONC intraocular injections with the antagonist were performed with a heat pulled glass pipette connected to a microsyringe (model 105; Drummond Microdispenser) 30 minutes after ONC. Intraocular injections were made via the dorsal limbus, each over a period of 1 min under anaesthesia (ketamine 50 mg/kg–rompun 10 mg/kg, i.p.).

ICON

Detection of retrogradely labelled RGCs was performed by using the ICON-method to show the same cells in vivo at various time points. The imaging was performed as previously described [28]. Briefly, animals were deeply anaesthetized with a mixture (3 ml/kg body weight i.m.) of ketamine (100 mg/ml), xylazine (20 mg/ml), and acepromazine (20 mg/ml) before the eye was treated with Neosynephrine-POS 5% (Ursapharm, Saarbrücken, Germany) for relaxation of the iris. Vidisic optical gel (M. Pharma, Berlin, Germany) was applied as an immersion medium for the contact lens and for prevention of drying of the cornea. The rats were then positioned underneath a standard confocal laser scanning microscope (Odyssey-XL, Noran Instruments GmbH, Bruchsaal, Germany) with a large probe space and long working distance objective lens. The left or right eye, containing the fluorescently labelled RGCs, was positioned directly underneath the objective lens.

Calcium activity of the RGCs was determined as relative fluorescence intensity presented with a false colour system of the Intervision software package (Intervision, Noran Instruments GmbH). 2 μl Oregon Green BAPTA (diluted 1 to five in 0.1 M PBS pH 7.4) mounted on a glass slide was used as positive standard value (100%).

Tissue preparation for immunohistochemistry

After an appropriate survival time animals received a lethal dosis of Chloralhydrat (7% in 0.9% saline, 12 ml/kg body weight) and were transcardially perfused with 0.9% saline followed by an fixative mixture containing 4% paraformaldehyde, 15% satured picric acid, 0.1% glutaraldehyde in 0.1 M phosphate-buffer pH 7.4. Optic nerves were removed from the skull and postfixed in glutaraldehyde-free fixative for additional 2 h and were processed further for immunohistochemistry. Therefore, the tissues were dehydrated in a graded series of ethanol, and embedded in Epon 812. Semithin longitudinal or transversal sections of the optic nerves were cut at 0.5 μm and mounted on microscopic slides.

Antisera

Polyclonal antisera anti-Neurofilament 200 (rabbit, 1:1000, Sigma, Deisenhofen, Germany) was used. Secondary Antibodies (1:50) were conjugated with FITC or Cy3 (anti-rabbit or anti-mouse, Sigma). Controls were carried out by omitting the first or second antibody.

Immunohistochemistry

After removal of Epon 812 by immersion for 2 min in sodium methoxide [13] the slides were incubated for 12 h at room temperature (RT) with the first antisera in 0.1 M PBS containing 0.1% BSA and 0.5% Tween 20. Between the various steps of the staining protocol the slides were thoroughly rinsed in 0.01 M PBS, pH 7.4.

Fluorescence microscopy

The tissue sections were examined with a fluorescence microscope (Leitz DM RXE) provided with a CCD camera (Kappa type CF8/4DXC, Kappa Opto-electronics GmbH, Gleichen, Germany). Software of Kappa ImageBase Control 2.0 (Kappa Opto-electronics GmbH) and Photoshop (version 5.0, Adobe Systems, Edinburgh, UK) were used for computerized imaging of the pictures.

Statistical analysis of optic nerve sections immunoreactive for NF-H

Pictures of longitudinal sections of the optic nerves stained with the NF-H antiserum were counted independently by two examiners. The counting parameters for the longitudinal sections were as follows: length of stained individual axons and their appearance as straight or wavelike. At the time points investigated (21 days after ONC with and without nifedipine injections, and sham-operated controls) four cases were measured and counted. In each case eight

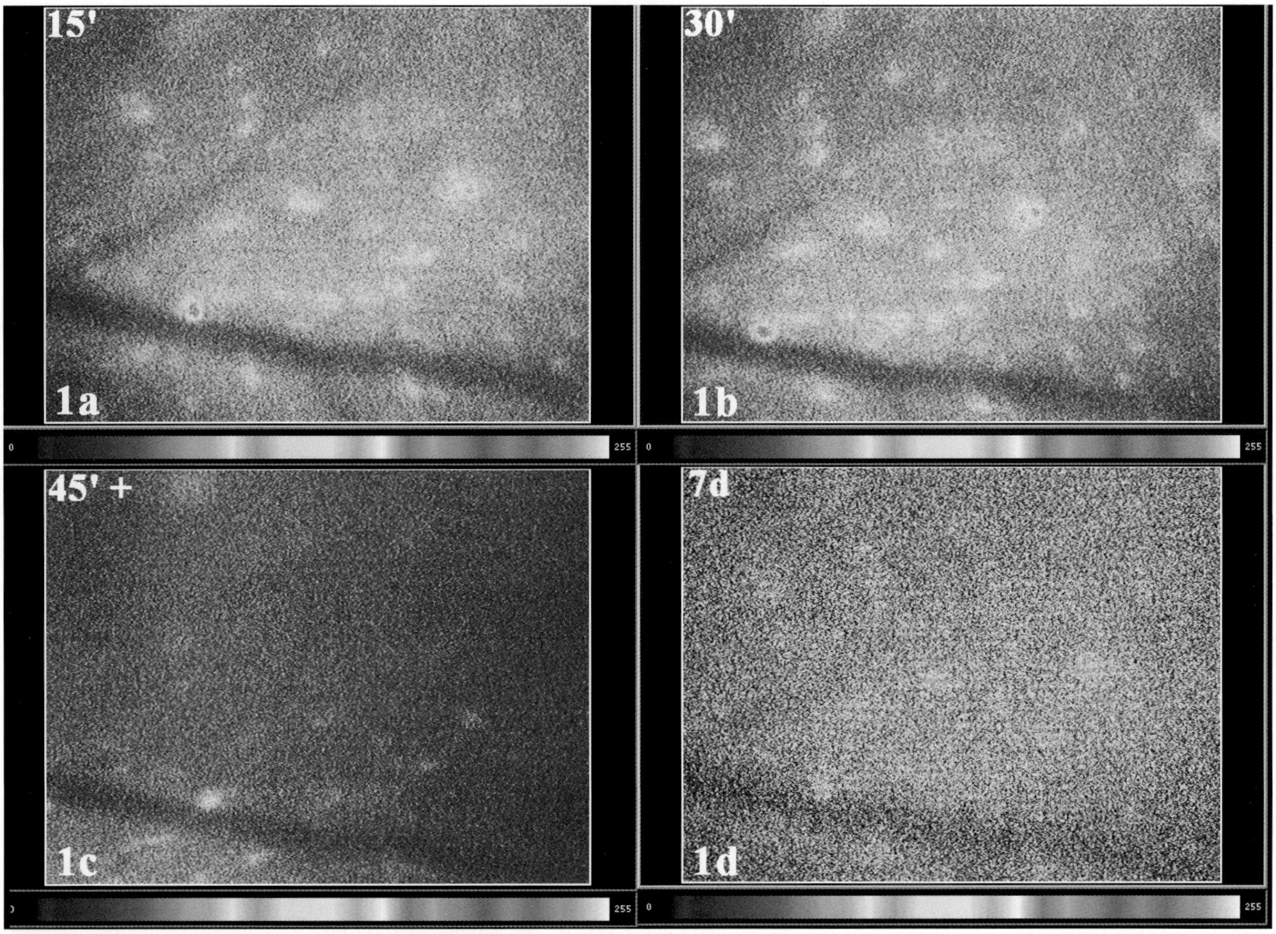

Fig. 1. Detection of RGCs after ONC with the ICON-method. The cells were retrogradely labelled with the fluorescence marker Oregon Green BAPTA to represent relative calcium activity as false colours (white respected to the highest calcium activiy and black to the lowest one). (a) Representation of RGCs with increased calcium activity 15 minutes after ONC. (b) Some RGCs increased further in fluorescence intensity 30 minutes after ONC. (c) After intraocular injection of the L-type calcium channel antagonist nifedipine most of the cells decreased rapidly in calcium activity. (d) At day 7 after ONC very few RGCs are visible in the same retina as (a–c). High background staining indicated an outflow of the fluorescence marker maybe by necrotic cell death

or nine pictures from different sections were analysed. After confirming time point-related differences of the stained axons with a non-parametric Kruskal-Wallis one-way ANOVA, a Dij-Test (based on differences between the rank sums of the groups) was performed for multiple comparisons.

Results

Calcium activity after ONC

The calcium activity of the RGCs was investigated with the ICON method using the fluorescent calcium marker Oregon Green BAPTA to determine possible changes after ONC. 15 min after ONC retrogradely labelled RGCs were recognized by their bright fluorescence of the calcium marker Oregon Green BAPTA (Fig. 1a). 30 min after ONC the relative calcium activity in the some cells was upregulated and soma size increased (Fig. 1b). Intraocular application of the L-type calcium channel antagonist nifedipine decreased rapidly the calcium activity in the RGCs as it was shown in fig. 1c. 7 days after ONC very few RGCs were visible. High background staining of the fluorescence marker indicated leakage of the Oregon Green probably as a consequence of necrotic cell death (Fig. 1d). After 3 weeks almost no staining of the RGCs was visible (results not shown). These RGCs disappeared from the image presumably because they have died.

Table 1. *Kruskal-Wallis one-way ANOVA results of two independent examiners, which counted axonal segments, stained for NF-H in longitudinal sections*

Axon length, appearance	First examiner			Second examiner		
	DF	Chi-square	p	DF	Chi-square	p
<2.75 μm, wavelike	5	13.80	n.s.	5	30.76	$p < 0.05$
<2.75 μm, straight	5	28.90	$p < 0.01$	5	20.50	$p < 0.01$
<8.25 μm, wavelike	5	20.76	n.s.	5	34.39	$p < 0.01$
<8.25 μm, straight	5	16.49	n.s.	5	32.54	$p < 0.01$
<16.5 μm, wavelike	5	18.36	n.s.	5	26.54	n.s.
<16.5 μm, straight	5	37.52	$p < 0.01$	5	37.49	$p < 0.005$
>16.5 μm, wavelike	5	23.15	n.s.	5	11.00	n.s.
>16.5 μm, straight	5	37.79	$p < 0.005$	5	41.04	$p < 0.005$

Immunohistochemistry

NF-H immunoreactivity in the axon fibers of the optic nerve showed statistically significant differences (Kruskal-Wallis one-way ANOVA between the groups) in axonal morphology in longitudinal sections 21 days after ONC, 21 days after ONC and application of nifedipine, and controls (Table 1). 21 days after ONC and application of nifedipine axonal segments stained for NF-H were shorter and displayed more swellings (Fig. 2a) as compared to the controls ($p < 0.01$ in the Dij-test based on differences between the rank sums of the groups) and the group untreated with nifedipine ($p < 0.05$, Dij-test). In the ONC group without nifedipine treatment the number of axons stained for NF-H decreased but most axonal segments stained for NF-H were straight and longer at day 21 (Fig. 2b) similar to the neurofilaments stained in the control sections (Fig. 2c). Thus, the percentage of long axonal segments (more than 16.5 μm) stained for NF-H at day 21 without further treatment was not significantly different from control sections. At day 21 after ONC and application of nifedipine a marked decrease of long axonal segments stained for NF-H was observed ($p < 0.01$ as compared to controls and $p < 0.05$ for day 21 ONC only, Dij-test). This showed a decrease of longer and straight axonal segments stained for NF-H at day 21 after ONC and a single injection for nifedipine as compared to the restitution

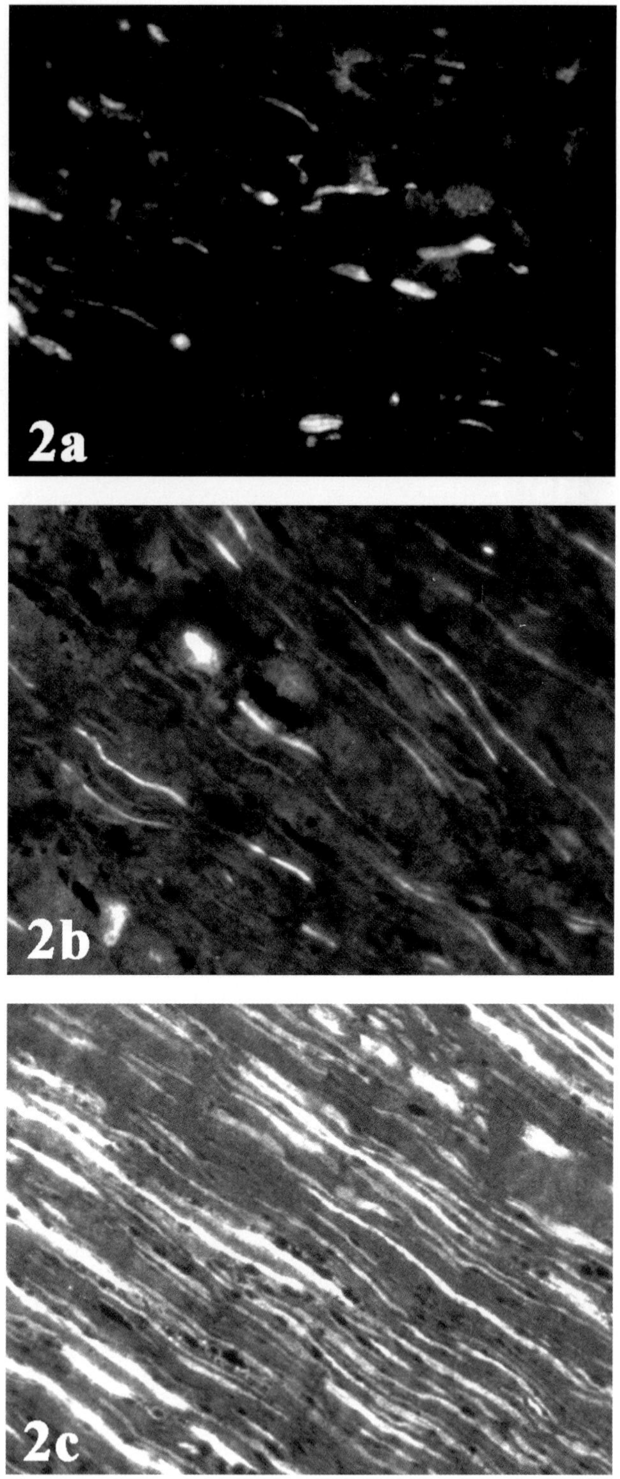

Fig. 2. Immunoreactive NF-H was detected in axon fibers of the optic nerve in longitudinal semithin sections. (a) At day 21 after ONC and intraocular injection of the L-type calcium channel antagonist nifedipine short fragments are mostly stained for NF-H in the axons. (b) At day 21 after ONC without any further modifications, few straight and longer axonal segments stained for NF-H. This indicates the normal restitution of the axon skeleton after optic nerve injury. (c) Control section stained for NF-H. Note the different diameters of the axon fibers

of the axonal skeleton, which was visible 21 days after ONC only.

Discussion

Using the ICON method in combination with an intracellular calcium marker and immunofluorescence for NF-H it was shown in the present investigation that restitution of NF-H in the injured optic nerve within 3 weeks after DAI was reduced strongly by a single injection of the L-type calcium channel antagonist nifedipine short after ONC.

Calcium dextran markers have been used successfully for investigation of neuronal activity [14, 16]. The strong dependence of the fluorescent signal on cell activity suggests that the technique is useful for monitoring the activity of identified neuronal populations [18]. With such a marker it was possible to detect qualitative and quantitative differences in calcium activity by measuring changes in fluorescence intensity in the RGCs with the ICON-method.

It is known that opening of voltage-dependent calcium channels contributes largely to intracellular calcium overload during excitotoxic events or following axon injury. Glutamate-mediated depolarization leads to activation of voltage-dependent calcium channels, allowing extracellular calcium to enter the cell along its concentration gradient. Therefore, an antagonist of L-type calcium channels, Nimodipine, has been evaluated in controlled randomised trials for neuroprotection in acute ischemia using various treatment regimens. The Intravenous Nimodipine West European Stroke Trial (INWEST) had to be terminated due to worsened outcome and increased mortality [1]. Another study, with patients who had been given nimodipine orally, found a significant 38% reduction of the odds for an unfavourable outcome only in those patients who had received the treatment within the first 12 h after the onset of symptoms [17]. The early treatment approach is now being tested in a Dutch study (Very Early Nimodipine Use in Stroke, VENUS; Limburg 1996). Thus, in the present study another antagonist of the L-type calcium channel, the clinically used nifedipine, was applicated. It was also injected 30 min after ONC to prevent rapid calcium induced swelling of about 65% of the total RGCs which undergo cell death shortly after ONC [26]. In another study, observation of surviving RGCs after ONC showed a modulatory and temporally delayed increase of intracellular calcium and cell soma size after 6 days [25, 26]. This protective calcium increase was not observed at day 7 in the present study after a single injection of nifedipine shortly after ONC. This indicates that the decision wether the cell will survive or undergo cell death is made very early after optic nerve injury.

Following ONC there is an initial period of necrotic and apoptotic RGC cell death [3] accompanied by complete blindness. Using different methods (immunofluorescence, functional tracing, ICON method, RT-PCR) it was shown that recovery of visual function correlates with the restitution of the cytoskeleton and the axonal transport in the injured optic nerve 3 weeks after DAI [8].

Calcium mediated injury is known to disrupt the neurofilaments within the axonal cytoskeleton [32] and calcium influx after experimental brain injury activates intracellular proteases like calpain leading to breakdown products of NF-H and NF-L in cortical tissue [20]. But, as it is shown here, an intracellular calcium decrease shortly after ONC did not result in restitution of the axonal cytoskeleton indicating that the calcium influx in this time window is critical for the recovery of neurones after DAI. The re-occurrence of straight NF-H in surviving axons 21 days after ONC (Fig. 2b) suggested an intrinsic axon repair in concert with the recovery of axonal transport and the restitution of vision [8].

Restoration of NF composition seems to play a crucial role in intrinsic axon repair as a requirement of recovery of vision [7]. The availability of NFs depends on its phosphorylation state and this state is under control of the modulatory effect of calcium [10]. Therefore a fine adjustment of calcium influx is necessary. A modulatory concert of different ion channels has to be created, a requirement that is not met by a nifedipine treatment shortly after DAI.

Acknowledgment

Supported by grants from the Deutsche Forschungsgemeinschaft (DFG, Sa 433/10-1) and the Ministery of Education and Research (BMBF, Neurotraumaverbund Magdeburg/Berlin, A2 FKZ: 01KO9813). We thank K. Hahn and S. Matzke for administrative assistance. The skillful technical assistance of Mrs A. Schulze is gratefully acknowledged.

References

1. Ahmed N, Nasman P, Wahlgren NG (2000) Effect of intravenous nimodipine on blood pressure and outcome after acute stroke. Stroke 31: 1250–1255
2. Berridge MJ, Bootman MD, Lipp P (1998) Calcium – a life and death signal. Nature 395: 645–648

3. Bien A, Seidenbecher CI, Bockers TM, Sabel BA, Kreutz MR (1999) Apoptotic versus necrotic characteristics of retinal ganglion cell death after partial optic nerve injury. J Neurotrauma 16: 153–163
4. Chesnut RM, Carney N, Maynard H, Mann NC, Patterson P, Helfand M (1999) Summary report: evidence for the effectiveness of rehabilitation for persons with traumatic brain injury. J Head Trauma Rehabil 14: 176–188
5. Duvdevani R, Rosner M, Belkin M, Sautter J, Sabel BA (1990) Graded crush of the rat optic nerve as a brain injury model: combining electrophysiological and behavioral out-come. Restor Neurol Neurosci 2: 31–38
6. Gennarelli TA, Adams JH, Graham DI (1986) Diffuse axonal injury. A new conceptual approach to an old problem. In: Baetmann A, Go, Unterberg A (eds) Mechanisms of secondary brain damage. Plenum, New York, pp 15–28
7. Hanke J, Schröder U, Sabel BA (2000) Internal axon repair after optic nerve crush in adult rats. Rest Neurol Neurosci 16: 225
8. Hanke J, Schröder U, Nahmmacher V, Sabel BA (2001): Repair of internal axon damage following traumatic optic nerve injury. Ann Anatomy [Suppl] 183
9. Hossmann KA, Paschen W, Csiba L (1983) Relationship between calcium accumulation and recovery of cat brain after prolonged cerebral ischemia. J Cereb Blood Flow Metab 3: 346–353
10. Julien JP, Mushynski WE (1998) Neurofilaments in health and disease. Prog Nucleic Acid Res Mol Biol 61: 1–23
11. Kasten E, Wuest S, Sabel BA (1998) Residual vision in transition zones in patients with cerebral blindness. J Clin Exp Neuropsychol 20: 581–598
12. Maxwell WL, Povlishock JT, Graham DL (1997) A mechanistic analysis of nondisruptive axonal injury: a review. J Neurotrauma 14: 419–440
13. Mayor HD, Hampton JC, Rosario B (1961) A simple method for removing the resin from epoxy embedded tissue. J Cell Biol 9: 909–910
14. McClellan AD, McPherson D, O'Donovan MJ (1994) Combined retrograde labelling and calcium imaging in spinal cord and brainstem neurons of the lamprey. Brain Res 663: 61–68
15. McKerracher L, Hirscheimer A (1992) Slow transport of the cytoskeleton after axonal injury. J Neurobiol 23: 568–578
16. McPherson DR, McClellan AD, O'Donovan MJ (1997) Optical imaging of neuronal activity in tissue labeled by retrograde transport of Calcium Green Dextran. Brain Res 1: 157–164
17. Mohr JP, Mast H, Thompson JL, Sacco RL (1998) Are more complex study designs needed for future acute stroke trials? Cerebrovasc Dis 8 [Suppl] 1: 17–22
18. O'Donovan MJ, Ho S, Sholomenko G, Yee W (1993) Real-time imaging of neurons retrogradely and anterogradely labelled with calcium-sensitive dyes. J Neurosci Methods 46: 91–106
19. Pantoni L, Garcia JH, Gutierrez JA (1996) Cerebral white matter is highly vulnerable to ischemia. Stroke 27: 1641–1646
20. Posmantur R, Hayes RL, Dixon CE, Taft WC (1994) Neurofilament 68 and neurofilament 200 protein levels decrease after traumatic brain injury. J Neurotrauma 11: 533–545
21. Povlishock JT, Erb DE, Astruc J (1992) Axonal response to traumatic brain injury: reactive axonal change, deafferentation, and neuroplasticity. J Neurotrauma 9 [Suppl] 1: S189–S200
22. Povlishock JT, Christman CW (1995) The pathobiology of traumatically induced axonal injury in animals and humans: a review of current thoughts. J Neurotrauma 12: 555–564
23. Povlishock JT, Marmarou A, McIntosh T, Trojanowski JQ, Moroi J (1997) Impact acceleration injury in the rat: evidence for focal axolemmal change and related neurofilament sidearm alteration. J Neuropathol Exp Neurol 56: 347–359
24. Raghupathi R, McIntosh TK (1998) Pharmacotherapy for traumatic brain injury: a review. Proc West Pharmacol Soc 41: 241–246
25. Rousseau V, Engelmann R, Sabel BA (1999) Restoration of vision III: soma swelling dynamics predicts neuronal death or survival after optic nerve crush in vivo. Neuroreport 10: 3387–3391
26. Rousseau V, Tietgens H, Rohatgi T, Hanke J, Sabel BA (2000) Adaptive versus lethal calciumactivity rise in retinal ganglion cells after optic nerve crush. Rest Neurol Neurosci 16: 66
27. Saatman KE, Graham DI, McIntosh TK (1998) The neuronal cytoskeleton is at risk after mild and moderate brain injury. J Neurotrauma 15: 1047–1058
28. Sabel BA, Engelmann R, Humphrey MF (1997a) In vivo confocal neuroimaging (ICON) of CNS neurones. Nature Med 3: 244–247
29. Sabel BA, Kasten E, Kreutz MR (1997b) Recovery of vision after partial visual system injury as a model of post-lesion neuroplasticity. Adv Neurol 73: 251–276
30. Sautter J, Sabel BA (1993) Recovery of brightness discrimination in adult rats despite progressive loss of retrogradely labelled retinal ganglion cells after controlled optic nerve crush. Europ J Neurosci 5: 680–690
31. Simon RP, Griffiths T, Evans MC, Swan JH, Meldrum BS (1984) Calcium overload in selectively vulnerable neurons of the hippocampus during and after ischemia: an electron microscopy study in the rat. J Cereb Blood Flow Metab 4: 350–361
32. Waxman SG, Black JA, Ransom BR, Stys PK (1993) Protection of the axonal cytoskeleton in anoxic optic nerve by decreased extracellular calcium. Brain Res 614: 137–145

Correspondence: Dr. Joachim Hanke, Institute of Anatomy, Medical Faculty, Otto-von-Guericke University, Leipzigerstrasse 44, D-39120 Magdeburg, Germany. e-mail: Joachim.Hanke@medizin.uni-magdeburg.de

Acta Neurochir (2004) [Suppl] 89: 81–85

Printed in Austria

Neuronal activity and cortical perfusion determined by quantitative EEG analysis and laser Doppler flowmetry are uncoupled in brain injured rats

J. F. Stover, O. W. Sakowitz, and **A. W. Unterberg**

Charité-Department of Neurosurgery, Berlin, Germany

Summary

Following traumatic brain injury uncoupling of metabolism from perfusion, reflected by an increase in cellular activity in face of reduced perfusion contributes to secondary tissue damage.

Standard autoradiographic techniques employed to study metabolism and perfusion are limited by the inability to perform longitudinal investigations. Therefore, the aims of this study were to investigate if metabolic uncoupling can be studied by applying non-invasive and non-radioactive methods. For this, quantitative EEG analysis and laser Doppler flowmetry were employed to determine changes in EEG activity as a global measure of neuronal activity and pericontusional cortical perfusion during the early phase following controlled cortical impact injury (CCII).

In eight rats changes in neuronal activity and pericontusional cortical perfusion were determined before, at 4 and 24 hours after CCII.

Neuronal activity was significantly increased by 40% at 4 hours after CCII followed by a significant decrease by 60% at 24 hours compared to pre-trauma levels. Pericontusional cortical perfusion was significantly reduced by 45% and 18% at 4 and 24 hours after CCII, respectively.

Non-radioactive methods like quantitative EEG analysis and laser Doppler flowmetry can be used to reveal underlying uncoupling of EEG activity from cortical perfusion which is mostly sustained in the early phase following CCII.

Keywords: Cortical perfusion; neuronal activity; secondary injury; traumatic brain injury.

Introduction

Under physiological conditions neuronal activity influences cerebral perfusion to meet elevated energetic demands [4]. Sustained release and changes in different mediators as e.g., potassium, nitric oxide, pCO_2, pH, calcium, adenosine, adenine nucleotides, neurotransmitters, and prostaglandins [6] are known to decrease cerebrovascular tone, thereby dilating cerebral arterioles and increasing cerebral blood flow. Under pathological conditions following ischemic [1, 17] and traumatic brain injury [5, 9], and during epileptic activity [2], however, metabolism and cerebral blood flow are no longer coupled. In this state of uncoupling cellular activity exceeds cerebral perfusion resulting in a mismatch between metabolism and supply of required energetic compounds. During the early posttraumatic period different pathological changes occur in parallel, develop sequentially and influence each other. In this regard, reduced cerebral perfusion due to platelet accumulation, leukocyte plugging, microcirculatory stasis, arteriolar vasoconstriction, edema-mediated compression of capillaries, and disturbed autoregulation [6] aggravate ongoing metabolic and energetic impairment as reflected by increased extracellular glutamate, lactate, and hypoxanthine concentrations [14]. Metabolic uncoupling is accepted to contribute to evolving secondary injury during the early period following ischemic and traumatic brain injury.

Investigation of uncoupling is usually performed by standard autoradiographic techniques [1, 5, 9]. However, injection of radioactive markers does not allow to perform longitudinal studies. Therefore, the aim of the present work was to determine if uncoupling of metabolism from blood flow can be monitored using non-invasive and non-radioactive methods. For this, changes in EEG activity as a global measure of neuronal activity and cellular metabolism were assessed by quantitative electroencephalographic recordings and local pericontusional cortical perfusion was investigated by laser Doppler flowmetry before trauma, at 4 and 24 hours following focal cortical contusion in the same rats.

Materials and methods

Controlled cortical impact injury (CCII)

Under isoflurane anesthesia (isoflurane: 1.6 vol%, N_2O: 0.4 l/min, O_2 0.2 l/min) CCII was induced by accelerating a pneumatic impactor (diameter 5 mm; penetration depth 1 mm, velocity 7 m/sec) in 10 male Sprague Dawley rats (300–350 g). This resulted in a significant left temporoparietal contusion and brain edema as recently published [18].

Physiological parameters

Mean arterial blood pressure (MABP) and arterial blood gases were determined before CCII, at 4 and 24 hours after trauma (table 1). Rectal temperature was maintained between 37 and 38 °C using a homeothermic heating pad.

Electroencephalographic recordings (EEG)

Two Ag/AgCl electrodes were attached to the exposed skull bone (right parietal and left frontal region) and referenced to the tail. EEG signals were amplified and digitized using a custom-built system. To avoid electrical interference a 50 Hz notch filter was applied. Wideband filtered data was sampled at 1 kHz and recorded on a PC-computer system. Off-line signal analysis in terms of quantitative EEG was performed using an automated artifact rejection algorithm on 1-minute epochs. Spectral power was calculated from artifact-free epochs using a Hanning-window prior to the Fast Fourier Transformation. Only the most dominant coefficients (1–3 Hz, δ power) reflecting cortical neuronal activity were assessed and expressed in μV^2.

Cortical perfusion

Pericontusional cortical perfusion was measured by laser Doppler flowmetry (DRT4, Moor Instruments, England) as described previously [10]. In brief, a 0.8 mm needle probe was moved in 40 × 0.2 mm steps over the brain surface of the traumatized hemisphere parallel to the sagittal suture and parallel to the contusion. Using the coordinates of the stereotaxic frame identical areas were investigated at different time points. Two scans were performed at each investigated time point requiring an average time of 9 minutes per scan. Cortical perfusion assessed by laser Doppler flowmetry is expressed as changes in percent to pre-trauma levels.

Statistical analysis

Results are presented as mean ± SEM. Parameters were compared for significant differences using one-way analysis of variances (ANOVA). Differences were rated significant at $p < 0.05$.

Results

Physiological parameters

During the entire study period arterial blood gases and MABP remained within physiological limits (Table 1).

Table 1. *Arterial blood gases and mean arterial blood pressure (MABP) remained stable during the entire study period*

	Before CCII	4 hours	24 hours
MABP [mmHg]	90 ± 1	92 ± 1	95 ± 3
pH	7.45 ± 0.01	7.45 ± 0.01	7.46 ± 0.02
$paCO_2$ [mmHg]	37.5 ± 1.9	36.1 ± 1.7	35.3 ± 1.6
paO_2 [mmHg]	174 ± 7	168 ± 12	203 ± 7
SBC [mmol/l]	26.4 ± 0.6	25.4 ± 0.5	26.3 ± 0.3
Hb [g/dl]	14.2 ± 0.3	13.2 ± 0.6	13.2 ± 0.8

EEG activity

Exemplary recordings of EEG activity (raw data) determined before, at 4 and 24 hours after CCII are depicted in Fig. 1 showing an increase in burst-density at 4 hours after trauma. Compared to pre-trauma levels EEG power was significantly increased at 4 hours followed by a significant reduction at 24 hours after CCII (Fig. 2).

Pericontusional cortical perfusion

At 4 hours after CCII pericontusional cortical perfusion was significantly decreased followed by an increase in flow values approaching pre-trauma levels at 24 hours (Fig. 2).

Uncoupling

Uncoupling, defined as an increase in metabolism as reflected by sustained EEG activity coinciding with decreased perfusion is found during the early phase, i.e., 4 hours following CCII (Fig. 2). Persisting severe functional disturbance is revealed by a significant reduction in EEG power despite nearly normalized flow values at 24 hours.

Discussion

Focal cortical contusion is associated with increased EEG activity and reduced pericontusional cortical perfusion during the early posttraumatic phase, possibly reflecting uncoupling of metabolism/neuronal activity from blood flow. These observed changes depict local cerebral disturbances which are not caused by systemic alterations since MABP, $paCO_2$, and hemoglobin count remained unchanged and within normal limits.

Compared to standard autoradiographic techniques [1, 5, 9] use of quantitative EEG and laser Doppler

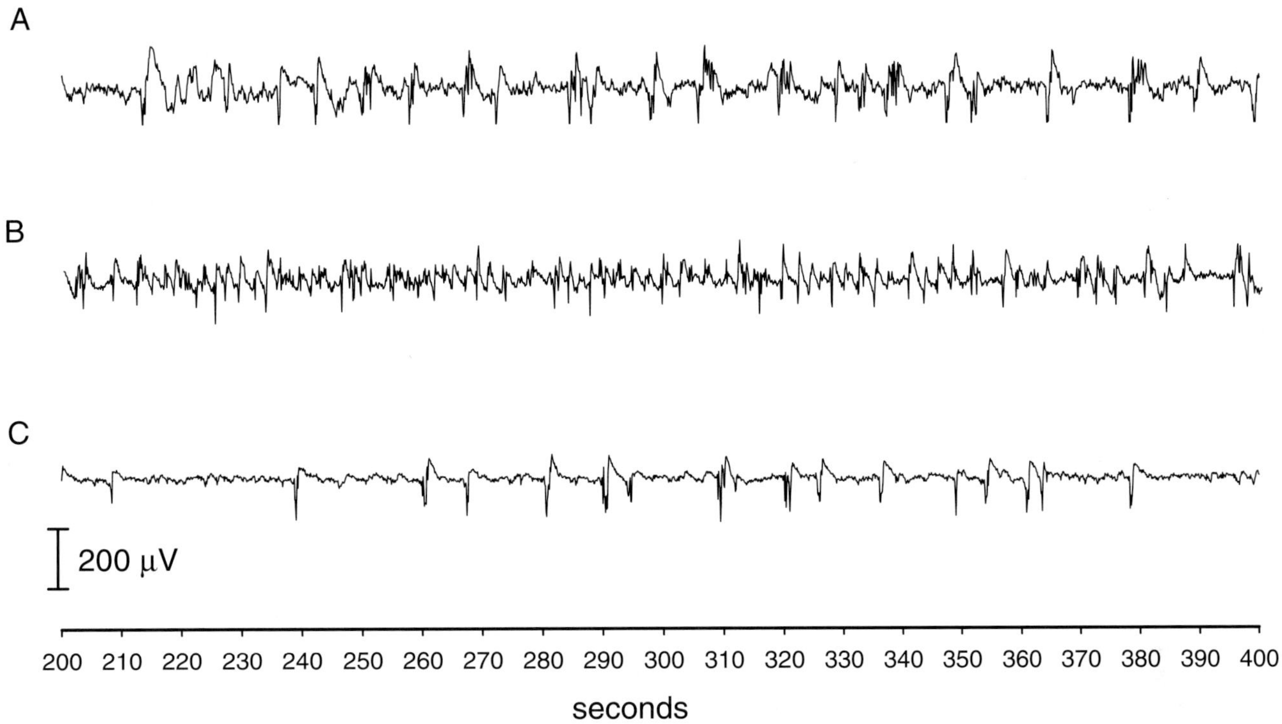

Fig. 1. Original EEG tracings determined before CCII (A), at 4 hours (B), and 24 hours (C) after CCII. Ordinate is given in μV. Abscissa in seconds

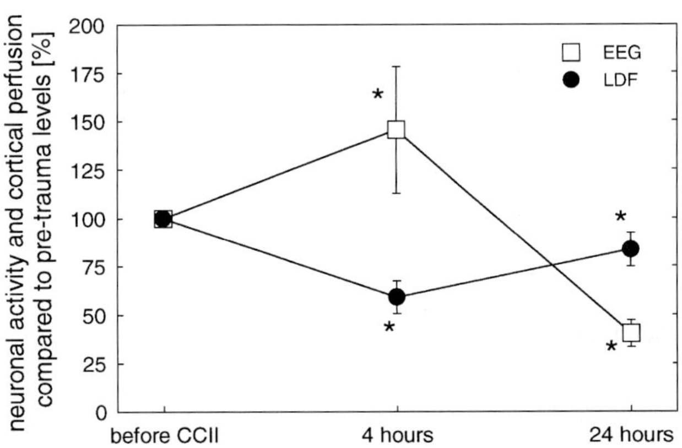

Fig. 2. Changes in EEG activity and pericontusional cortical perfusion determined by quantitative EEG analysis and laser Doppler flowmetry *(LDF)*, respectively are expressed in percent to pre-trauma levels. Following CCII EEG activity was significantly increased at 4 hours followed by a significant decrease at 24 hours (*$p < 0.05$, ANOVA). Cortical perfusion was significantly decreased, which was mostly sustained at 4 hours after CCII (*$p < 0.05$, ANOVA)

flowmetry analysis to determine changes in global neuronal activity and pericontusional cortical blood flow, respectively allow to conduct longitudinal studies.

Employing the scanning technique by moving a laser Doppler probe in defined steps using the coordinates of the stereotaxic frame allows to assess local changes in pericontusional cortical perfusion. However, EEG analysis and laser Doppler flowmetry cannot be used to topographically map changes in cellular activity and perfusion in different regions at varying depths of the rat brain as in autoradiography.

Using a second laser Doppler probe for the contralateral hemisphere would allow to simultaneously assess changes in the traumatized and non-traumatized hemisphere. However, alterations within deeper structures as e.g., the hippocampus known for its sustained vulnerability to glutamate-mediated excitation can only be visualized autoradiographically.

Due to its high temporal resolution EEG analysis is particularly useful in studying functional changes that lead to alterations in cortical excitatory and inhibitory postsynaptic potentials. Spatial resolution, however, is usually poor. This can be partially solved by, e.g., using grid electrodes to obtain multi-channel recordings.

Assessment of spectral band-power as performed in the present study can be used to quantitate EEG activity in the anesthetized rat. This, in turn allows to study functional disturbance of neuronal networks following traumatic brain injury [21].

Posttraumatic hyperglycolysis is caused by sustained neuronal and glial activation [5]. Autoradiographic studies do not allow to differentiate between neuronal and glial activation while EEG analysis can be used to explicitly investigate changes in neuronal activity. Sustained activation of postsynaptic glutamate receptors and energy-requiring pumps, as e.g., the Na^+/K^+ ATPase result in increased glucose metabolism and lactate production which can be reduced by NMDA and non-NMDA receptor antagonists [8]. Disturbance of ionic homeostasis and development of spreading depression-like depolarizations following ischemic and traumatic brain injury stimulate glucose utilization [1, 5]. These depolarizations linked to increased activity of energy-consuming pump processes coincide with attenuated perfusion, thereby aggravating energetic impairment and contributing to cellular damage. Over time, depolarizations increase in duration and are accompanied by a reduction in EEG amplitude [1]. At 24 hours after CCII, neuronal activity determined by quantitative EEG analysis was decreased in amplitude and frequency. This decrease in neuronal activity is in line with depressed glucose utilization in contused cortex and ipsilateral subcortical regions between 1 and 10 days following CCII [9, 19]. It remains to be clarified if a mere loss in cortical neurons linked to a reduction in neuronal excitation or if functional disturbance in terms of spreading depression-like depolarizations account for the reduction in EEG power.

Among other targets, the volatile anesthetic isoflurane attenuates neuronal activity by reducing presynaptic glutamate release [11] and interfering with postsynaptic glutamate receptor binding [12] in a concentration-dependent fashion [16]. To exclude any artificial changes in EEG activity rats were anesthetized with identical isoflurane concentrations, i.e., 1.6 vol% at all investigated time points. However, it remains to be clarified if the susceptibility of neurons to the anesthetic action of isoflurane changes over time, thereby contributing to the observed temporal profile of neuronal activity. In the early phase, i.e., 1 to 12 hours following ischemia NMDA and non-NMDA-receptor-mediated excitatory postsynaptic currents were significantly enhanced in hippocampal neurons [13]. Therefore, the administered isoflurane concentration could have been too low to reduce neuronal activity at 4 hours after CCII while theoretically the same concentration could have been too high in relative terms, thereby significantly reducing neuronal activity at 24 hours after CCII, a time point characterized by a marked loss in cortical neurons.

Seizure activity occurs within the early period following traumatic brain injury under experimental [15] and clinical conditions [20]. Using the chosen setup we cannot exclude occurrence of non-convulsive epileptic activity in the early phase following CCII, possibly contributing to the increase in EEG power.

Reduction in perfusion observed in the early phase following CCII is caused by structural and functional disturbances involving endothelial cells, thrombocytes, leukocytes and humoral factors. As determined by intravital microscopy (unpublished data) and described by other authors, arteriolar vasoconstriction, platelet aggregation, leukocyte plugging, resulting in microvascular stasis, contribute to significant flow reduction. In addition, an imbalance between dilating (nitric oxide) and constricting (endothelins) factors gives rise to diminished perfusion [6].

Pathophysiologic features of metabolic uncoupling can be influenced pharmacologically [7] and by moderate hypothermia [3], resulting in a decrease in tissue damage. It remains to be clarified if specific inhibition of presynaptic glutamate release and elevation in MABP as performed in clinical routine via continuous norepinephrine infusion can be used to reduce EEG activity and increase cerebral perfusion, respectively, thereby modulating uncoupling of cellular activity from perfusion and possibly reducing secondary tissue injury.

References

1. Back T, Zhao W, Ginsberg MD (1995) Three-dimensional image analysis of brain glucose metabolism-blood flow uncoupling and its electrophysiological correlate in the acute ischemic penumbra following middle cerebral artery occlusion. J Cereb Blood Flow Metab 15: 566–577
2. Bruehl C, Hagemann G, Witte OW (1998) Uncoupling of blood flow and metabolism in focal epilepsy. Epilepsia 39: 1235–1242
3. Chen Q, Choppp M, Bodzin G, Chen H (1993) Temperature modulation of cerebral depolarization during focal cerebral ischemia in rats: correlation with ischemic injury. J Cereb Blood Flow Metab 13: 389–394
4. Ginsberg MD, Smith DW, Wachtel MS, Gonzalez-Carvajal M, Busto R (1986) Simultaneous determination of local cerebral glucose utilization and blood flow by carbon-14 double-label autoradiography: method of procedure and validation studies in the rat. J Cereb Blood Flow Metab 6: 273–285
5. Ginsberg MD, Zhao W, Alonso OF, Loor-Estades JY, Dietrich WD, Busto R (1997) Uncoupling of local cerebral glucose metabolism and blood flow after acute fluid-percussion injury in rats. Am J Physiol 272: H2859–H2868

6. Golding EM, Robertson CS, Bryan RM (1999) The consequences of traumatic brain injury on cerebral blood flow and autoregulation: a review. Clin Exp Hypertension 21: 299–332
7. Iijima T, Mies G, Hossmann K-A (1992) Repeated negative DC deflections in rat cortex following middle cerebral artery occlusion are abolished by MK-801: effect on volume of ischemic injury. J Cereb Blood Flow Metab 12: 727–733
8. Kawamata T, Katayama Y, Hovda DA, Yoshino A, Becker DP (1992) Administration of excitatory amino acid antagonists via microdialysis attenuates the increase in glucose utilization seen following concussive brain injury. J Cereb Blood Flow Metab 12: 12–24
9. Kelly DF, Kozlowski DA, Haddad E, Echiverri A, Hovda DA, Lee SM (2000) Ethanol reduces metabolic uncoupling following experimental head injury. J Neurotrauma 17: 261–272
10. Kroppenstedt SN, Stover JF, Unterberg AW (2000) Effects of dopamine on posttraumatic cerebral blood flow, brain edema, and cerebrospinal fluid glutamate and hypoxanthine concentrations. Crit Care Med 28: 3792–3798
11. Liachenko S, Tang P, Somogyi GT, Xu Y (1999) Concentration-dependent isoflurane effects on depolarization-evoked glutamate and GABA outflows from mouse brain slices. Br J Pharmacol 127: 131–138
12. MacIver B, Mikulec AA, Amagasu SM, Monroe VA (1996) Volatile anesthetics depress glutamate transmission via presynaptic actions. Anesthesiology 85: 823–834
13. Mitani A, Namba S, Ikemune K, Yanase H, Arai T, Kataoka K (1998) Postischemic enhancements of N-Methyl-D-Aspartic Acid (NMDA) and non-NMDA receptor-mediated responses in hippocampal CA1 pyramidal neurons. J Cereb Blood Flow Metab 18: 1088–1098
14. Nilsson P, Hillered L, Pontén U, Ungerstedt U (1990) Changes in cortical extracellular levels of energy-related metabolites and amino acids following concussive brain injury. J Cereb Blood Flow Metab 10: 631–637
15. Nilsson P, Ronne-Engström E, Flink R, Ungerstedt U, Carlson H, Hillered L (1994) Epileptic seizure activity in the acute phase following cortical impact trauma in rat. Brain Res 637: 227–232
16. Patel PM, Drummond JC, Cole DJ, Goskowicz RL (1995) Isoflurane reduces ischemia-induced glutamate release in rats subjected to forebrain ischemia. Anesthesiology 82: 996–1003
17. Singh NC, Kochanek PM, Schiding JK, Melick JA, Nemoto EM (1992) Uncoupled cerebral blood flow and metabolism after severe global ischemia in rats. J Cereb Blood Flow Metab 12: 802–808
18. Stover JF, Schoning B, Beyer TF, Woiciechowsky C, Unterberg AW (2000) Temporal profile of cerebrospinal fluid glutamate, interleukin-6, and tumor necrosis factor-alpha in relation to brain edema and contusion following controlled cortical impact injury in rats. Neurosci Lett 288: 25–28
19. Sutton RL, Hovda DA, Adelson PD, Benzel EC, Becker DP (1994) Metabolic changes following cortical contusion: relationships to edema and morphologic changes. Acta Neurochiur (Wien) [Suppl] 60: 446–448
20. Vespa PM, Nuwer MR, Nenov V, Ronne-Engström E, Hovda DA, Bergsneider M, Kelly DF, Martin NA, Becker DP (1999) Increased incidence and impact of nonconvulsive and convulsive seizures after traumatic brain injury as detected by continuous electroencephalographic monitoring. J Neurosurg 91: 750–760
21. West M, Parkinson D, Havlicek V (1982) Spectral analysis of the electroencephalographic response to experimental concussion in the rat. Electroenceph Clin Neurophysiol 53: 192–200

Correspondence: John F. Stover, M.D., Charité-Department of Neurosurgery, Augustenburger Platz 01, 13353 Berlin, Germany. e-mail: stoverfam@bluewin.ch

Acta Neurochir (2004) [Suppl] 89: 87–92

Printed in Austria

Glial scar and axonal regeneration in the CNS: lessons from GFAP and vimentin transgenic mice

M. G. Ribotta, V. Menet, and **A. Privat**

INSERM U, Université Montpellier, Cedex, France

Summary

Astrocytes play an active role in the brain and spinal cord. For example, they have a function in formation and maintenance of the blood-brain barrier, ion homeostasis, neurotransmitter transport, production of extracellular matrix, and neuromodulation. Moreover, they play a role in preserving or even restoring the structural and physiological integrity after tissue injury. Currently, the function of astrocytes was studied with regard to the controversially discussed aspects of permissivity on the one-hand-side and inhibition of the other side exerted by reactive astrocytes for axonal regrowth in the adult CNS. Accordingly, knock-out mice deficient in vimentin (VIM) and/or glial fibrillary acidic protein (GFAP), the two major IF-proteins of astrocytes, were investigated. In addition, in vitro studies were carried out, on whether the absence of one or both proteins (VIM, GFAP) influences axonal regeneration. In experimental animals, a hemisection of the spinal cord was performed utilizing the above mentioned double-mutant mice. The knock-out mice were generated by gene targeting. Double-mutants were obtained by crossing single null mice.

The in vitro results indicate that both VIM and GFAP were absent in astrocytic cultures obtained from double-mutant mice. On the other side, the proteins were detected in more than 85% of cultured cells from wild types. Co-culture of mutant mice astrocytes with neurons revealed that the neuronal density was different from that obtained in culture with wild type astrocytes. On the other side, there was a marked increase in neuronal density in co-cultures utilizing both GFAP knock-out- or double-mutant mice astrocytes again as compared to co-cultures with wild type astrocytes. Moreover, the neurite length of neurons was significantly increased in experiments with neurons growing on astrocytes from GFAP-knock-out or double-mutant mice.

The in vivo experiments demonstrate an increase of nestin (NES) immunoreactivity at three days in the sectioned side of the spinal cord, in the perikaryon and astroglial processes. In double-mutant mice only a slight increase in NES-immunoreactivity was found in the lesion side, albeit confined to the perikaryon of astrocytes. Below the lesion, serotonin immunostaining was dramatically reduced three days after the insult in both sides, particularly in the lesion side. The decrease was more pronounced in double-mutant than in wild type mice. On the other side, double-mutant mice had a much higher density of serotonergic fibers in the ventral horn in the lesioned side.

In conclusion, the findings demonstrate that in the absence of important astrocytic proteins as VIM and GFAP, the astroglial response to injury is significantly modified underlying reduced scar formation. Attenuation of scar formation may enhance axonal sprouting of serotonergic axons below the lesion, which specifically reinnervate motoneuron pools.

Keywords: Astrocyte/neuronal co-culture; axonal regeneration; vimentin; glial fibrillary acidic protein; knock-out mice; spinal cord hemisection.

Introduction

In the developing CNS, astrocytes have been shown to play a role as a structural substrate for neuronal migration and axonal elongation [38, 47]. In the mature CNS, astrocytes play an active role in integrative functions of the brain and spinal cord. Indeed, astrocytes participate in the formation and maintenance of the blood-brain barrier [54], ion homeostasis [52], neurotransmitter transport [45], production of extracellular matrix [19, 25], and neuromodulation [11, 32].

Moreover, astrocytes play a major role in preserving and restoring some degree of structural and physiological integrity following injury [42]. The astrocytic response to injury is characterized by the hyperplasia and hypertrophy of cell bodies and processes. These two parameters characterize the reactive gliosis which has been regarded as the major obstacle to the axonal regeneration and CNS repair [4, 22, 39, 42, 50]. In any case, the major hallmark of reactive gliosis is an up-regulation of two major intermediate filaments (IF) proteins of the astrocyte, vimentin (VIM) and glial fibrillary acidic protein (GFAP) [1, 7, 15, 35, 40]. An increase in GFAP mRNA levels at the lesion site is followed by the long term rise in GFAP immunoreactivity whereas a long term decrease in mRNA occurs [30, 41, 46]. A similar regulation of GFAP mRNA is also observed at distance from the lesion site, in the projection areas [40, 41, 51]. After injury, the reexpression of VIM occurs in astrocytes close to the injury and at distance from the lesion site in a subset of astrocytes associated with Wallerian degeneration [7, 29, 44].

In addition, reactive astrocytes also reexpress other IF class VI-protein, such as Nestin (NES) [5, 10, 21], which is predominantly expressed by neuroepithelial progenitor cells [8, 18]. NES is down-regulated in the adult CNS with the exception of adult CNS stem cells [16, 24, 31, 43, 53]. NES is also reexpressed in deafferented target territories [3]. Thus, like VIM and GFAP, NES constitutes a sensitive marker of reactive gliosis following CNS injury [3, 5, 10, 21].

However, the formation of the glial barrier at the lesion site has also positive aspects, such as the production of trophic factors [33], and an isolating role in reconstructing the blood-brain barrier (BBB), thus limiting secondary lesions.

This study reports our recent advances concerning the controversial aspects of permissivity and inhibition by reactive astrocytes for axonal regrowth in the adult CNS. After a previous study in which we used a cholesterol derivative to modify both the physical and chemical components of the astroglial barrier [13], we proposed to evaluate selectively the contribution of hypertrophy in the glial scar. For this purpose we used transgenic mice deficient in VIM or/and GFAP, the two major IF-proteins of the astrocyte involved in hypertrophic response to injury. We have investigated in vitro whether the absence of one or both proteins – VIM and GFAP – may influence axonal regeneration by modifying the surface properties and diffusible and/or matrix-associated factors of astrocytes, in terms of their ability to support neuronal survival or/and neurite outgrowth. We then analyzed in vivo the astroglial reaction and axonal regrowth in a hemisection model of the spinal cord using these double mutant mice.

Materials and methods

VIM-null and GFAP-null mice were generated by gene-targeting as previously described [6, 37]. Double mutant mice were obtained by crossing single null mice. Wild-type mice with a mixed genetic background were used in this study. We performed two experimental approaches: (1) an in vitro coculture model of neurons/astrocytes, and (2) an in vivo hemisection model of the spinal cord.

In vitro approach

Our purpose was to analyze the surface properties and diffusible or/and matrix-associated molecules of astrocytes from the three mutant mice with regard to neuronal survival and neuritogenesis, and to compare them to those from wild-type mice. We developed a coculture model using neonatal spinal cord astrocytes (P-2) from wild-type or mutant mice which reached confluence after 15 days in vitro (DIV), when embryonic cortex neurons (E-14) from wild-type mice were added. Such a coculture model permits the development of neurons on a well defined astrocyte monolayer from their target region. The same protocol was carried out with the three mutant mice.

Primary cultures of astrocytes were established from spinal cord as previously described [28]. Briefly, spinal cords were aseptically isolated and the meninges discarded. After treatment with 0.25% trypsin-EDTA for 8 min at 37 °C, tissue was mechanically dissociated, resuspended in a 1:1 mixture of Dulbecco's modified essential medium and Ham's F12 supplemented with 10% fetal bovine serum and 0.6% glucose, and plated at a final concentration of 10^5 cells/cm^2. After 15 days in vitro, cultured astrocytes attained confluence. Embryonic cortical neurons were prepared in the same way as astrocytes and seeded on astrocyte monolayers at the density of 12.5×10^3 cells/cm^2. Coculture medium was supplemented with N2 complement and changed every 3 days.

After 7 days in vitro, cocultured neurons were processed for βIII-tubulin immunodetection and two parameters were evaluated: neuronal survival and neurite lenghts per neuron. Some cultures with astrocytes alone were also characterized at 21 days in vitro by immunocytochemical detection of VIM, GFAP and NES, using the peroxidase-antiperoxidase system [27].

In vivo approach

Our aim in this approach was to analyze the astroglial reaction to injury in these mutant mice. Here we have evaluated astroglial response in double VIM and GFAP knockout mice using a previously described hemisection model of the spinal cord [13]. Then, axonal sprouting or regeneration was evaluated in these mutants versus wild-type mice. This hemisection model includes in addition an internal control by comparison of injured and intact sides in the same animal.

Following 3 days or 5 weeks to the lesion, animals were sacrificed by intracardial perfusion, spinal cords removed and processed for NES, S-100 immunodetection. Moreover, serotonergic sprouting was subsequently evaluated by immunocytochemistry [26].

Results

In vitro approach

Astrocyte monolayers

VIM, GFAP and NES were immunodetected in more than 85% of the cultured cells from wild-type mice. As expected, VIM and GFAP, respectively were absent in cultures from VIM and GFAP mutant mice, whereas both proteins were absent in cultures from double mutant mice. NES was normally expressed in cultures from GFAP mutant mice with a distribution similar to that of cultures from wild-type mice. However, in cultures from double mutant mice, NES immunostaining distribution appeared diffusely spread out in the perikaryon and no NES-immunoreactivity

Table 1. *Quantification of neuronal density and neurite length per neuron on astrocyte monolayers from wild-type, Vim-, GFAP- and double mutant mice after 7 days in vitro of coculture*

	Wild-type	Vim−/−	GFAP−/−	Double−/−
Neuronal density (cells/mm^2)	35.23 ± 5.92	24.60 ± 2.63	106.14 ± 14.81***	125.83 ± 16.76***
Neurite length (μm/neuron)	483.87 ± 40.19	531.40 ± 65.87	1125.86 ± 82.18***	1061.26 ± 78.68***

Values are indicated as absolute values ± *sem* and statistical analysis was performed using the non parametric Mann-Whitney U test (***: $p < 0.001$).

Neuronal density and total neurite length of wild-type neocortical neurons co-cultured on spinal cord astrocytes from VIM mutant mice do not significantly differ from that growing on astrocytes from wild-type mice. At variance, note the significant increase of both neuronal density and neurite length when neurons are cocultured on astrocytes from GFAP- and from double mutant mice.

was detected on astroglial processes whereas two astrocyte populations were detected in cultured astrocytes from VIM mutant mice: one with NES-network of glial filaments and the other with a diffuse pattern.

Cocultures

After characterization of cocultured neurons by βIII-tubulin immunostaining, two parameters were evaluated. *Neuronal density* for determining the influence of the absence of VIM or/and GFAP on neuronal attachment and survival, and *neurite length per neuron* for determining the influence of the VIM or/and GFAP on neurite growth.

Cortical neurons growing on astrocytes from wild-type mice appeared isolated and developed short neurites. A very similar aspect was observed when neurons grew on astrocytes from VIM mutant mice. In contrast, cortical neurons growing on astrocytes from both GFAP and double mutant mice were often organized in clusters, more so in the case of GFAP mutant mice, and both developed a long and more complex neuritic network.

Neuronal density in cocultures from VIM mutant mice was not significantly different from that of wild-type mice. Interestingly in contrast, a marked increase in neuronal density was observed in cocultures from both GFAP and double mutant mice versus cocultures from wild-type mice (Table 1).

The measure of neurite length per neuron permitted the evaluation of the efficacy of differential surface properties of astrocytes from these three mutant mice as regards neurite elongation. Neurite lengths per neuron in cultures from VIM mutant mice were not significantly different from those of wild-type mice. Conversely, neurite length per neuron in the case of neurons growing on astrocytes from both GFAP- and double mutant mice was significantly higher than that of neurons growing on astrocytes from wild-type mice (Table 1).

In vivo approach

In wild-type animals NES-immunoreactivity was increased as early as 3 days in the sectioned side in the perikaryon and astroglial processes and was still present at least 5 weeks after the hemisection of spinal cord. Conversely, in double mutant mice, a slight increase in NES-immunoreactivity was detected in the lesioned side, which was only confined to the perikaryon of astrocytes.

Below the lesion level, serotonin immunostaining was dramatically reduced 3 days after the lesion on both sides, but especially on the lesioned side. This reduction was more marked in double mutant than in wild-type mice. Five weeks after the lesion, a few thin serotonergic fibers were observed throughout the lesioned side in wild-type animals, whereas a much higher density of fibers concentrated in the ventral horn on the lesioned side was observed in double mutant mice.

Discussion

Our results illustrate several interesting points: First, VIM- or GFAP-immunostaining, like that observed in normal cultured astrocytes from wild-type mice, were observed in astrocytes respectively devoid of GFAP and VIM. No evident signs of compensatory expression of the partner IF-protein were observed in astrocytes devoid of VIM or GFAP, confirming the in vivo studies carried out by ourselves and others [12, 14, 37]. Secondly, normal distribution of NES immunoreactivity was only observed in astrocytes devoid of GFAP whereas a polymerized NES network was absent in astrocytes from VIM and double mutant mice. This confirms that NES needs the presence of VIM to polymerize in a NES/VIM network [9, 23] and not that of GFAP.

Moreover, our results show that astrocytes from GFAP- and double mutant mice are significantly more permissive for both neuronal survival and neurite outgrowth, at variance with astrocytes devoid of VIM which are more comparable to astrocytes from wild-type mice. Thus, the absence of GFAP in astrocytes (from both GFAP and double mutant mice) seems to be a key factor in the modification of neuron/astrocyte interactions, leading to a more favourable and permissive substrate for survival and neurite growth.

The increased neuronal survival observed on astrocytes devoid of GFAP or of both VIM and GFAP could be a consequence either of a better attachment of cortical neurons by increasing adhesive properties, or of a release of trophic factors. Moreover, astrocytes devoid of GFAP or both VIM and GFAP are a more permissive substrate for neurite growth, possibly by expression of diffusible or/and matrix-associated molecules in an increased permissive/inhibition ratio [20, 34]. The absence of GFAP could thus correspond in some aspects to a status close to that of radial glia, which contain only VIM and possibly NES, and which are permissive for migration and axonal elongation of neurons during development [38, 47, 48, 55] or similar to immature astroglia which are a more permissive substrate for neurite outgrowth than the mature astrocytes [2, 15, 49]. Interestingly, increased neurite outgrowth promoted by astrocytes from GFAP mutant mice [27] has also recently been obtained in neuron/astrocyte coculture by using GFAP m-RNA antisens [17].

The possible mechanisms involved in the effects of astrocytes devoid of GFAP (from GFAP and double mutant mice) are analyzed through the comparative screening of key molecules in three mutant and wild-type mice [28].

This study illustrates also that in the absence of VIM and GFAP, the two major IF-proteins of astrocytes, a significant modification of the parameters of astroglial reaction to injury occurs, leading to a reduced glial scar in the spinal cord which has been illustrated in another lesion model [36]. Moreover, this results in axonal sprouting of serotonergic axons below the lesion, which reinnervate specifically motoneuron pools.

Conclusion

Astrocytes are the indispensable partners of neurons, from birth to senescence. The progressive elucidation of their multiple functions opens-up new avenues for intervention in many pathological processes. One key example is indeed that of axonal regeneration where they appear as one of the main targets for drugs, cell and gene therapy. However, posttraumatic reaction of astrocytes illustrates the intricacy of protective/obstructive influences, whose complexity reflects that of the CNS of mammals. Ontogeny and phylogeny converge towards the most sophisticated assembly of living cells, which are all interdependent, and it should be remembered that any intervention in the complex cascade of events which follows an injury should be tailored in order to keep that assembly as intact as possible. Hopefully, we have now in our hands an equally sophisticated arsenal of diagnostic and therapeutic tools limited only by our imagination ...

Acknowledgments

We thank Dr. Colucci-Guyon and Dr. Babinet for valuable discussions, J. R. Teilhac for photographic works. This study was supported by grants from IRME, AFM, VERTICALE and BIOMED.

References

1. Bignami A, Dahl D (1976) The astroglia response to stabbing. Immunofluorescence studies with antibodies to astrocyte-specific protein (GFA) in mammalian and submammalian vertebrates. Neuropathol Appl Neurol 2: 99–111
2. Bovolenta P, Liem RK, Mason CA (1984) Development of cerebellar astroglia: transitions in form and cytoskeletal content. Dev Biol 102: 248–259
3. Brook GA, Perez-Bouza A, Noth J, Nacimiento W (1999) Astrocytes re-express nestin in deafferented target territories of the adult rat hippocampus. Neuroreport 10: 1007–1011
4. Brown JO, McCough GP (1947) Abortive regeneration of the transected spinal cord. J Comp Neurol 87: 131–137
5. Clarke SR, Shetty AK, Bradley JL, Turner DA (1994) Reactive astrocytes express the embryonic intermediate neurofilament nestin. Neuroreport 5: 1885–1888
6. Colucci-Guyon E, Portier MM, Dunia I, Paulin D, Pournin S, Babinet C (1994) Mice lacking vimentin develop and reproduce without an obvious phenotype. Cell 79: 679–694
7. Dahl D, Bignami A, Weber K, Osborn M (1981) Filament proteins in rat optic nerves undergoing Wallerian degeneration: localization of vimentin, the fibroblastic 100-A filament protein, in normal and reactive astrocytes. Exp Neurol 73: 496–506
8. Dahlstrand J, Lardelli M, Lendahl U (1995) Nestin mRNA expression correlates with the central nervous system progenitor cell state in many, but not all, regions of developing central nervous system. Dev Brain Res 84: 109–129
9. Eliasson C, Sahlgren C, Berthold CH, Stakeberg J, Celis JE, Betsholtz C, Eriksson JE, Pekny M (1999) Intermediate filament protein partnership in astrocytes. J Biol Chem 274: 23996–24006

10. Frisén J, Johansson CB, Török C, Risling M, Lendahl U (1995) Rapid, widespread, and longlasting induction of nestin contributes to the generation of glial scar tissue after CNS injury. J Cell Biol 131: 453–464
11. Fróes MM, Campos de Carvalho AC (1998) Gap junction-mediated loops of neuronal-glial interaction. Glia 24: 97–107
12. Giménez y Ribotta M, Langa F, Menet V, Privat A (2000) Comparative anatomy of the cerebellar cortex in mice lacking Vimentin, GFAP, and both Vimentin and GFAP. Glia 31: 69–83
13. Giménez y Ribotta M, Rajaofetra N, Morin-Richaud C, Alonso G, Bochelen D, Sandillon F, Legrand A, Mersel M, Privat A (1995) Oxysterol (7β-hydroxycholesteryl-3-oleate) promotes serotonergic reinnervation in the lesioned rat spinal cord by reducing glial reaction. J Neurosci Res 41: 79–95
14. Gomi H, Yokoyama T, Fujimoto K, Ikeda T, Katoh A, Itoh T, Itohara S (1995) Mice devoid of the glial fibrillary acidic protein develop normally and are susceptible to scrapie prions. Neuron 14: 29–41
15. Hatten ME, Liem RKH, Shelanski ML, Mason CA (1991) Astroglia in CNS injury. Glia 4: 233–243
16. Johansson CB, Momma S, Clarke DL, Risling M, Lendahl U, Frisén J (1999) Identification of a neural stem cell in the adult mammalian central nervous system. Cell 96: 25–34
17. Lefrançois T, Fages C, Peschanski M, Tardy M (1997) Neuritic outgrowth associated with astroglial phenotypic changes induced by antisense glial fibrillary acidic protein (GFAP) mRNA in injured neuron-astrocyte cocultures. J Neurosci 17: 4121–4128
18. Lendahl U, Zimmerman LB, McKay RD (1990) CNS stem cells express a new class of intermediate filament protein. Cell 60: 585–595
19. Liesi P, Dahl D, Vaheri A (1983) Laminin is produced by early rat astrocytes in primary culture. J Cell Biol 96: 920–924
20. Liesi P, Silver J (1988) Is astrocyte laminin involved in axon guidance in the mammalian CNS? Dev Biol 130: 774–785
21. Lin RCS, Matesic DF, Marvin M, McKay RD, Brüstle O (1995) Re-expression of the intermediate filament nestin in reactive astrocytes. Neurobiol Dis 2: 79–85
22. Liuzzi FJ, Lasek RJ (1987) Astrocytes block axonal regeneration in mammals by activating the physiological stop pathway. Science 237: 642–645
23. Marvin NJ, Dahlstrand J, Lendahl U, McKay RDG (1998) A rod end deletion in the intermediate filament protein nestin alters its subcellular localization in neuroepithelial cells of transgenic mice. J Cell Sci 111: 1951–1961
24. McKay R (1997) Stem cells in the central nervous system. Science 276: 66–71
25. McKeon RJ, Hoke A, Silver J (1995) Injury-induced proteoglycans inhibit the potential for laminin-mediated axon growth on astrocytic scars. Exp Neurol 136: 32–43
26. Menet V, Colucci-Guyon E, Babinet C, Privat A, Giménez y Ribotta M (1998) Astroglial and axonal responses to spinal cord injury in mice deficient for glial fibrillary acidic protein (GFAP) and Vimentin (VIM). Abs Soc Neurosci 710: 6
27. Menet V, Giménez y Ribotta M, Sandillon F, Privat A (2000) GFAP null astrocytes are a favourable substrate for neuronal survival and neurite growth. Glia 31: 267–272
28. Menet V, Giménez y Ribotta M, Chavet N, Drian MJ, Lannoy J, Colucci-Guyon E, Privat A (2001) Inactivation of the glial fibrillary acidic protein gene, but not that of vimentin, improves neuronal survival and neurite growth by modifying adhesion molecule expression. J Neurosci 21: 6147–6158
29. Mikucki SA, Oblinger MM (1991) Vimentin mRNA expression increases after corticospinal axotomy in the adult hamster. Metab Brain Dis 6: 33–49
30. Morin-Richaud C, Feldblum S, Privat A (1998) Astrocytes and oligodendrocytes reactions after a total section of the rat spinal cord. Brain Res 783: 85–101
31. Morshead CM, Reynolds BA, Craig CG, McBurney MW, Staines WA, Morassutti D, Weiss S, Van der Kooy D (1994) Neural stem cells in the adult mammalian forebrain: a relatively quiescent subpopulation of subependymal cells. Neuron 13: 1071–1082
32. Nedergaard M (1994) Direct signaling from astrocytes to neurons in cultures of mammalian brain cells. Science 263: 1768–1771
33. Nieto-Sampedro M, Lewis ER, Cotman CW, Manthorpe M, Skaper SD, Barbin G, Longo FM, Varon S (1982) Brain injury causes a time-dependent increase in neuronotrophic activity at the lesion site. Science 271: 860–861
34. Noble M, FokSeang J, Cohen J (1984) Glia are a unique substrate for the in vitro growth of central nervous system neurons. J Neurosci 4: 1892–1903
35. Oblinger MM, Singh LD (1993) Reactive astrocytes in neonate brain upregulate intermediate filament gene expression in response to axonal injury. Int J Dev Neurosci 11: 149–156
36. Pekny M, Johansson CB, Eliasson C, Stakeberg J, Wallén A, Perlmann T, Lendahl U, Betsholtz C, Berthold CH, Frisén J (1999) Abnormal reaction to central nervous system injury in mice lacking glial fibrillary acidic protein and vimentin. J Cell Biol 145: 503–514
37. Pekny M, Leveen P, Pekna M, Eliasson C, Berthold CH, Westermark B, Betsholtz C (1995) Mice lacking glial fibrillary acidic protein display astrocytes devoid of intermediate filaments but develop and reproduce normally. EMBO J 14: 1590–1598
38. Rakic P (1995) Radial glial cells: Scaffolding for brain construction. In: Kettenmann H, Ransom BR (eds) Neuroglia. Oxford University Press, New York, pp 746–762
39. Ramón Y, Cajal S (1928) Degeneration and regeneration of the nervous system. In: May RM (ed) Oxford University Press, London
40. Rataboul P, Faucon Biguet N, Vernier P, De Vitry F, Boularand S, Privat A, Mallet J (1988) Identification of a human glial fibrillary acidic protein cDNA: a tool for the molecular analysis of reactive gliosis in the mammalian central nervous system. J Neurosci Res 20: 165–175
41. Rataboul P, Vernier P, Privat A (1990) Analysis of glial scarring in the mammalian CNS with a GFAP cDNA probe. In: Lauder JM, Privat A, Giacobini E, Timiras PS, Vernadakis A (eds) Molecular aspects of development and aging of the nervous system. Adv Exp Med Biol, vol 265. Plenum Press, New York, pp 23–40
42. Reier PJ, Eng LF, Jakeman L (1989) Reactive astrocyte and axonal outgrowth in the injured CNS: Is gliosis really an impediment to regeneration? In: Seil J (ed) Neural regeneration and transplantation, frontiers of clinical neuroscience, vol 6. Alan R Liss, Inc, New York, pp 183–209
43. Reynolds BA, Weiss S (1992) Generation of neurons and astrocytes from isolated cells of the adult mammalian central nervous system. Science 255: 1707–1710
44. Schiffer D, Giordana MT, Migheli A, Giaccone G, Pezzotta S, Mauro A (1986) Glial fibrillary acidic protein and vimentin in the experimental glial reaction of the rat brain. Brain Res 374: 110–118
45. Schousboe A, Westergaard N (1995) Transport of neuroactive amino acids in astrocytes. In: Kettenmann H, Ransom BR (eds) Neuroglia. Oxford University Press, New York, pp 246–258
46. Shafit-Zagardo B, Kume Iwaki A, Goldman JE (1988) Astrocytes regulate GFAP mRNA levels by cyclic AMP and protein kinase C-dependent mechanisms. Glia 1: 346–354

47. Silver J, Edwards MA, Levitt P (1993) Immunocytochemical demonstration of early appearing astroglial structures that form boundaries and pathways along axon tracts in the fetal brain. J Comp Neurol 328: 415–436
48. Singer M, Nordlander RH, Egar M (1979) Axonal guidance during embryogenesis and regeneration in the spinal cord of the newt: the blueprint hypothesis of neuronal pathway patterning. J Comp Neurol 185: 1–21
49. Smith GM, Rutishauser U, Silver J, Miller RH (1990) Maturation of astrocytes in vitro alters the extent and molecular basis of neurite outgrowth. Dev Biol 138: 377–390
50. Stensaas LJ, Partlow LM, Burgess PR, Horch KW (1987) Inhibition of regeneration: the ultrastructure of reactive astrocytes and abortive axon terminals in the transition zone of the dorsal root. In: Seil FJ, Herbert E, Carlson BM (eds) Neural regeneration, progress in brain research, vol. 71. Elsevier, Amsterdam, pp 457–467
51. Steward O, Kelley MS, Torre ER (1993) The process of reinnervation in the dentate gyrus of adult rats – Temporal relationship between changes in the levels of glial fibrillary acidic protein (GFAP) and GFAP mRNA in reactive astrocytes. Exp Neurol 124: 167–183
52. Walz W (1989) Role of glial cells in the regulation of the brain ion microenvironment. Prog Neurobiol 33: 309–333
53. Weiss S, Dunne C, Hewson J, Wohl C, Wheatley M, Peterson AC, Reynolds BA (1996) Multipotent CNS stem cells are present in the adult mammalian spinal cord and ventricular neuroaxis. J Neurosci 16: 7599–7609
54. Wolburg H, Risau W (1995) Formation of the blood-brain barrier. In: Kettenmann H, Ransom BR (eds) Neuroglia. Oxford University Press, New York, pp 763–776
55. Zheng C, Heintz N, Hatten ME (1996) CNS gene encoding astrotactin, which supports neuronal migration along glial fibers. Science 272: 417–419

Correspondence: Alain Privat, INSERM U. 336, Université Montpellier II, Place E. Bataillon, B.P. 106, 34095 Montpellier, Cedex 05, France. e-mail: u336@univ-montp2.fr

Traumatic brain and spinal cord injury – clinical progress including treatment

Acta Neurochir (2004) [Suppl] 89: 95–100

Printed in Austria

Recovery from spinal cord injury – underlying mechanisms and efficacy of rehabilitation

V. Dietz and **G. Colombo**

ParaCare, Swiss Paraplegic Centre of the University Hospital Bagrlist, Zurich, Switzerland

Summary

Patients with an acute complete spinal cord injury (SCI) present a syndrome called "spinal shock". During spinal shock the loss of tendon reflexes and flaccid muscle tone is associated with a low persistence of F-waves and loss of flexor reflexes while H-reflexes are well elicitable. When clinical signs of spasticity become established, the electrophysiological parameters show little change. The divergent course of clinical signs of spasticity in their possible neuronal correlates indicate the occurrence of non-neuronal changes contributing to spasticity. – When signs of spinal shock had disappeared in patients with incomplete and complete paraplegia a locomotor pattern can be induced and trained under conditions of body unlaoding using a moving treadmill. In complete and incomplete paraplegic patients an increase of gastrocnemius electromyographic activity occurs during the stance phase of a step cycle with a daily locomotor training, coincident with a significant decrease of body unloading. In contrast to this, neither clinical nor electrophysiological examination scores improve. The locomotor pattern depends on the level of lesion: the higher the level of spinal cord lesion the more 'normal' is the locomotor pattern. This suggests that neuronal circuits underlying 'locomotor pattern generation' in man is not restricted to any specific level of the spinal cord, but extends from thoraco-lumbal to cervical levels.

Keywords: Spinal cord injury; spinal shock; spasticity; locomotor training.

Introduction

The vertebrate CNS has a limited capacity for regeneration. Much of the research effort aimed at improving functional recovery after spinal cord injury is directed towards enhancing the limited ability of CNS neurones to restore damaged connections between the spinal cord and brain. After many SCI there is some preservation of anatomical continuity across the injury site, even in patients with minimal function below the lesion [1]. The problem then becomes one of maximizing the functional contribution of the preserved pathways and if axonal regeneration also becomes possible of newly regenerated projections.

After spinal cord injury, restoration of normal function, such as locomotion, will depend to a certain extent upon reorganization of existing spinal circuitry. This capacity for reoganization, generally referred to as plasticity, is a well-known property of the CNS, and is thought to underline many instances of functional recovery after injury, as well as learning and memory in the undamaged CNS. While plasticity has been well documented in many parts of the supraspinal CNS, the prevalent view of spinal cord function has been that it is relatively non-plastic and serves simply as a hard-wired relay for supraspinal commands. This view has been changing with the accumulation of physiological and behavioural evidence that adaptive processes can also occur within spinal circuits. The potential ability of the spinal cord to 'learn' has obvious implications for altering and improving locomotor function after injury.

The neural mechanisms responsible for learning and adaptive processes are thought to involve changes both in the efficacy of synaptic function and the pattern of synaptic connections within neural circuits. In the uninjured CNS, these changes occur as a result of alteration in the amount of neural activity within circuits and are therefore termed activity-dependent. After CNS injury, there also appears to be reorganization of spared neural circuits. The mechanisms underlying this injury-induced plasticity are not understood fully, although it is possible that some of these changes are also guided in an activity-dependent manner (for review see Muir and Steves [2]).

Spinal cord injury can produce a number of significant changes in the anatomy and physiology of spinal cord neuronal circuitries. Sprouting of spared axons is perhaps the best studied anatomical change after injury. In this instance, sprouting refers to the expansion of the terminal fields of undamaged axons when the terminals of injured axons degenerate. Although, there has been some controversy over the extent and conditions under which terminals sprouting takes place, results indicate that, caudal to a spinal hemisection in cats or monkeys, the central terminal projections of dorsal-root afferents can increase the density and extent of their distribution [3, 4, 5].

From spinal shock to spasticity

The clinical recovery from spinal shock is characterized by the re-appearance of tendon tap reflexes and of muscle tone. These clinical signs are reflected by a change in the excitability of neuronal correlates [6].

Clinical and neurophysiological background

More than 100 years ago the term "spinal shock" was introduced to describe the clinical state in patients with acute spinal cord injury (SCI) presenting muscle paralysis with flaccid muscle tone and loss of tendon reflexes below the level of lesion [7]. Although complete loss of sensorimotor function persists, spinal shock ends after some weeks and during the following months a "spastic syndrome" develops with exaggerated tendon reflexes, increased muscle tone and involuntary muscle spasms. The development of a spastic syndrome is a common finding in surgically or pathologically confirmed complete spinal cord transection [8], i.e. changes in the excitability of spinal cord neuronal circuits occur independently of supraspinal influences.

In order to explain these changes several hypothesis were put forward based on clinical observations, neurophysiological recordings, intracellular studies and theoretical considerations. A change from hypoexcitability of alpha-motoneurons (alpha-MN) during spinal shock to hyperexcitability during spasticity was presumed [9]. According to this concept the alpha-MN hypoexcitability in spinal shock is due to an acute loss of supraspinal excitatory input resulting in a hyperpolarized alpha-MN [10]. Such a hyperpolarization of spinal MN was observed in spinalized cats [11].

In contrast to this, well elicitable H-reflexes were described in humans early after SCI [12, 13] contradicting a strong alpha-MN depression as single cause for the loss of tendon tap reflexes during spinal shock. The latter observation led to the concept of concomitant gamma-motoneuron (gamma-MN) depression [13]: While a mechanical tap does not elicit a tendon tap reflex, electrical stimulation of group I afferent nerve fibers leads to a H-reflex response.

Furthermore interneuron (IN) activity and excitability has an important influence on spinal neuronal activity. It is known that most of the supraspinal descending tracts impinge on spinal interneurons [14]. An interruption of these tracts will influence spinal IN function. However, up to now little is known about the changes in IN activity that occur during spinal shock and the transition to spasticity.

Relationship between clinical and electrophysiological parameters

In the study of Hiersemenzel and coworkers [6] clinical and electrophysiological parameters were systematically assessed in patients after an acute SCI.

The period of spinal shock was electrophysiologically associated with a reduced excitability of alpha-MN reflected by a low persistence of F-waves, which is in line with previous studies [15, 16]. This observation may be related to the clinical signs found at this stage: the loss of tendon reflexes and muscle hypotonia. The neurophysiological basis of the reduced alpha-MN excitability may be due to the sudden loss of tonic input and/or trophic support from supraspinal to spinal neuronal centers. For instance, nor-adrenergic pathways were suggested to be responsible for the excitability level of alpha-motoneurons [17]. In view of other data on effects of serotonin (5-hydroxytryptamin; 5-HT) on spinal motoneurons, both 5-HT and other descending pathways might be involved as well (for review see [18]).

The results of the electrophysiological measurements in humans fit well with the data obtained in animal cellular recordings which show hyperpolarization of resting membrane potential [11, 19]. In the light of the close interaction between MN and muscle [20] the initial reduction of M-wave amplitude (described also in [13]) might be seen as a consequence of the changed MN behavior.

In contrast to the neuronal depression reported above, H-reflexes could be elicited already at an early stage after SCI, which is in accordance with earlier reports [9, 13] The discrepancy between preserved H-reflex and the loss of tendon reflexes as a typical clinical sign might at least partially be due to a reduced activity of gamma-MN. However, one has to keep in mind that the level of fusimotor drive is not the only factor affecting muscle spindle responsiveness [21].

Nevertheless, the early excitability of the H-reflex does not fit well with the assumption of an overall depression of neuronal activity including all motoneurons as a common final pathway of spinal neuronal activity. Several mechanisms could account for this discrepancy: First, the present observations are in line with the view described earlier for chronic paraplegic patients that presynaptic inhibition of group Ia-afferents is, at least partially, removed after SCI [22, 23]. Previous studies have shown a supraspinal influence on presynaptic inhibition of Ia-afferents [24]. The decrease in presynaptic inhibition may compensate for the decreased excitability of alpha-MN. Consequently, early after SCI up to the spastic state a maximal H-reflex may be obtained which overrides the decreased excitability of alpha-MN assessed by F-waves. Second, one has to keep in mind that F-waves are caused by backfiring of only about 1% of motoneurons [25] and that H-reflex and F-wave were not investigated in the same muscle. Therefore H-reflexes and F-waves may reflect the excitation of different populations of alpha-MN, which only partially overlap with the consequence that the excitability of the H-reflex does not parallel the persistence of the F-wave.

While H-reflex was present early and F-wave persistence was low (but usually F-waves could be recorded), there was a loss of flexor reflex activity in the TA early after SCI. The latter observation indicates a suppression of IN activity mediating this polysynaptic reflex (for review see [26]). However, we are aware that comparisons between the three types of responses have to be made with caution as they were obtained (for physiological reasons) from different leg muscles.

The recovery from spinal shock is reflected by an increase in the excitability of tendon tap reflexes and in muscle tone (assessed by the Ashworth scale) as well as more frequently occurring muscle spasms (assessed by the Penn spasm frequency scale). These clinical changes were associated in the electrophysiological recordings by an increase of F-wave persistence and flexor reflex activity [6]. There was only a minor change in H-reflex excitability during this time period. It may be suggested that the increase in tendon tap reflex excitability is at least partially due to a recovery of alpha-MN and probably also of gamma-MN function mediating this reflex.

The increase in flexor reflex activity should not only be due to a recovery of alpha-MN excitability, but also to the function of spinal interneuronal circuits (see spinal shock). The fact that the flexor reflex is more difficult to elicit in healthy subjects than in para-/tetraplegic patients [27] indicates an increased excitability of interneuronal circuits some weeks after SCI. The pathway underlying the flexor reflex is a polysynaptic spinal one and allows the integration of inputs from muscles, joints and cutaneous afferents on common interneurons (for review see [18]).

The changes in flexor reflex excitability may at least partly be reflected in the appearance of muscle spasms. The increase in muscle tone may be due to a more general recovery of spinal neuronal (alpha-MN and IN) activity. Nevertheless, for both clinical parameters reflecting recovery from spinal shock (Penn spasm frequency and Ashworth scale) it cannot be ruled out, that other factors than the neuronal activity recorded here, as well as changes of muscle biomechanics, contribute to the development of spasticity.

Clinically, the *development of the spastic syndrome* is characterized by exaggerated muscle tendon tap reflexes, increased muscle tone and involuntary muscle contractions. The onset of spastic signs is difficult to determine because there is a smooth transition to a clearly established spasticity.

During this stage, both M-wave and flexor reflex amplitudes remained about stable in tetraplegic or decreased in amplitude in paraplegic patients, i.e. developed even opposite to the clinical signs [6]. The slight increase of H/M-ratio, which is in line with an earlier study [22], might contribute to exaggerated tendon tap reflexes. However, this increase which was thought to be well correlated with the spastic state (for review [28]) must be considered cautiously: 1. The high H/M-ratio can express rather a decrease of M-wave (as found here) than an increase in reflex excitability. 2. Short latency reflex hyperexcitability was shown to be little related to spastic muscle tone [29].

On the basis of the observations made in the study of Hiersemenzel *et al.* [6] clinical signs of increasing spasticity, such as muscle tone and spasms, can hardly be related to the electrophysiological recordings. Secondary changes of motor units might contribute to the syndrome of spasticity, especially in respect to muscle tone and spasms.

Several studies claim that "peripheral changes" (e.g. chronic transformation of muscle in spasticity) contribute to the increased muscle tone [30, 31]. A decrease of M-wave in patients with a SCI [32] or those with a cerebral lesion [23] indicates an affection of spinal MN in the case of a disconnection from supraspinal input. Furthermore, signs of denervation are described to occur during the first 2 months after SCI [33]. It became obvious during the last years that following a central motor lesion changes in mechanical muscle fiber properties occur starting early after a lesion with the consequence of a significant contribution to muscle tone in the active (for review see [34]) and passive muscles ([35], for review see [29]).

Locomotor activity in spinal man

Evidence for a spinal locomotor pattern

Although there is strong evidence for a spinal locomotor generator in many mammals (for review see [36]), its existence has, until recently, been questioned in man [37]. Evidence for the human spinal pattern generator was suggested by spontaneously occurring step-like movements [38] and myoclonus [39] as well as from late flexion reflexes [40] and from locomotor movements induced on a treadmill with body support in paraplegic patients (for review see [36]). Recent studies showed that a locomotor pattern can be induced in complete paraplegic patients when leg movements were assisted from externally [41]. Nevertheless, the amplitude of leg muscle EMG activity in these patients was small compared to healthy subjects, (most probably due to the loss of noradrenergic influences from brainstem centres) such that no leg movements resulted from this leg muscle activation.

A recent study [42] has demonstrated that a locomotor pattern can only be induced some weeks after SCI, when spinal reflexes re-appear. The question, therefore, was to what degree the EMG pattern recorded may be due to the activity of spinal stretch reflexes as suggested elsewhere [43]. Correlation studies between leg muscle EMG activity and the lengthening and shortening phases of respective leg muscles (tibialis anterior and gastrocnemius) showed that leg muscle EMG activity is equally distributed during the lengthening and shortening phases of the respective leg muscles (tibialis anterior (TA) and gastrocnemius (GM)). For the GM it was taken into account, that this is a biarticulate muscle. In both the healthy subject and the paraplegic patient there was a near equal distribution of EMG activity during muscle stretch of these muscles in the stance and swing phases, respectively. An about equal distribution of EMG-activity was also found in all other patients.

The earliest time that spinal locomotor activity could be induced was when signs of spinal shock had disappeared. This activity was distinct from spinal stretch reflex activity. In complete paraplegic patients the locomotor pattern improved spontaneously without training [42]. This was coincident with both an increase of gastrocnemius electromyographic activity during the stance phase of gait and a decrease of body unloading. These effects reached a plateau after about 5 weeks.

Localization of the central pattern generator

In patients even with severe or complete paraplegia, coordinated leg muscle activation underlying stepping movements can be induced by partial body weight support concomitant with standing on a moving treadmill [41, 44, 45, 46, 47]. It remained unclear to what extent the level of lesion can influence the locomotor pattern and which part(s) of the spinal cord need to be preserved for locomotor pattern generation. From experiments in the cat there is evidence that the neuronal centres involved in locomotion are widespread within the spinal cord and the brainstem [17, 48]. However, this may be different in bipedal locomotion of human beings where the lumbosacral spinal cord contains the motoneurons supplying leg muscles.

The question remains which part of the spinal cord is responsible for or is involved in the generaton of the locomotor pattern. To answer this question, the locomotor pattern was analyzed in complete para-/tetraplegic patients with various levels of spinal cord lesion [49].

It was found that the locomotor neuronal circuits are not discrete, but that an intricate neuronal network of interconnected nerve cells up to at least cervical levels contributes to generation of increasingly complex human locomotor patterns. It cannot be decided from these observations in how far a widespread network as a whole generates the locomotor pattern or, alternatively, whether neuronal circuits within the lumbosacral spinal cord operate more effectively to induce locomotion when neurons in more rostral segments regulate their activity. Furthermore, in patients with a low spinal lesion a loss of trunk afferent input could lead to a reduced EMG amplitude.

Conclusions

Based on animal experiments recent investigations have shown that the isolated human spinal cord contains neuronal centres, which are able to generate complex movements. Nevertheless, the activation of these centres, with the aim to improve mobility of paraplegic patients, is still limited.

1. After an acute spinal cord injury (SCI) basic changes in the spinal neuronal activity takes place, which at part are associated with alterations of signs assessed by the clinical examination. The changes seen in the clinical signs from spinal shock to spasticity were shown to be only partially reflected by the neuronal correlates assessed by electrophysiological recordings, for example, when increased muscle tone becomes established and muscle spasms appear. The divergent course of clinical signs of spasticity and the probable neuronal correlates indicate the occurrence of non-neuronal changes contributing to spasticity. However, one has to be aware that at present we are able to evaluate only a part of the spinal neuronal activity.
2. Based on observations of the locomotor capacity of the spinal cat, recent studies have indicated that spinal locomotor centres can be activated and be trained in patients with complete or incomplete paraplegia, when the body is partially unloaded. The level of electromyographic activity (EMG) in the leg extensor muscles, however, is considerably lower in patients with central motor lesions than in person without neurological impairment. During the course of a locomotor training programme the amplitude of the EMG increases associated with an improvement of locomotor function in the patients. Only incomplete paraplegic patients profit from this training for their locomotor ability. Furthermore, there are also unspecific training effects on muscles and ligaments.
3. In complete para-/tetraplegic patients the level of lesion determines the locomotor activity in spinal man. The higher the level of spinal cord lesion the more "normal" is the locomotor pattern. This suggests that neuronal circuits underlying locomotor pattern generation extend form thoraco-lumbal to cervical levels. This observation may have important therapeutic implications in the future when it might become possible to induce some regeneration of spinal tract fibres.
4. In complete or almost complete paraplegic patients who at present do not yet profit from a locomotor training might profit in the near future from experimental therapies that facilitate regeneration of adult CNS axons. Potential therapeutic inverventions include growth promoting factors, such as bridging transplants and neutralisation of myelin-associated factors that inhibit axonal outgrowth.

Acknowledgments

This work was supported by the Intenational Institute for Research on Paraplegia (P49/99) and the Swiss National Research Foundation (No 31-53526.98).

References

1. Dimitrijevic MR (1988) Residual motor functions in spinal cord injury. Adv Neurol 47: 138–155
2. Muir GD, Steeves JD (1997) Sensorimotor stimulation to improve locomotor recovery after spinal cord injury [see comments]. Trends Neurosci 20: 72–77
3. Helgren ME, Goldberger ME (1993) The recovery of postural reflexes and locomotion following low thoracic hemisection in adult cats involves compensation by undamaged primary afferent pathways. Exp Neurol 123: 17–34
4. Goldberger ME, Murray M (1988) Patterns of sprouting and implications for recovery of function. Adv Neurol 47: 361–385
5. Goodman CS, Shatz CJ (1993) Developmental mechanisms that generate precise patterns of neuronal connectivity. Cell [Suppl] 72: 77–98
6. Hiersemenzel LP, Curt A, Dietz V (2000) From spinal shock to spasticity: neuronal adaptations to a spinal cord injury. Neurol 54: 1574–1582
7. Bastian HC (1890) On the symptomatology of total transverse lesions of the spinal cord, with special reference to the condition of the various reflexes. Med Chir Trans (Lond) 73: 151–217
8. Kuhn R (1950) Functional capacity of isolated human spinal cord. Brain 73: 1–51
9. Diamantopoulos E (1967) Excitability of motor neurones in spinal shock in man. J Neurol Neurosurg Psychiatry 30: 427–431
10. Ashby P, Verrier M, Lightfoot E (1974) Segmental reflex pathways in spinal shock and spinal spasticity in man. J Neurol Neurosurg Psychiatry 37: 1352–1360
11. Schadt JC, Barnes CD (1980) Motoneuron membrane changes associated with spinal shock and the Schiff-Sherrington phenomenon. Brain Res 201: 373–383
12. Leis AA, Zhou HH, Mehta M, Harkey HL, Paske WC (1996) Behavior of the H-reflex in humans following mechanical perturbation or injury to rostral spinal cord. Muscle Nerve 19: 1373–1382
13. Weaver R, Landau W, Higgins J (1963) Fusimotor function. Part 2: evidence of fusimotor depression in human spinal shock. Arch Neurol 9: 127–132
14. Baldissera F, Hultborn H, Illert M (1981) Integration in spinal neuronal system. In: The nervous system, motor control, vol 2, part 1. American Physiological Society, Washington, DC, pp 509–595
15. Curt A, Keck ME, Dietz V (1997) Clinical value of F-wave recordings in traumatic cervical spinal cord injury. Electroencephalogr Clin Neurophysiol 105: 189–193

16. Leis AA, Stetkarova I, Beric A, Stokic DS (1996) The relative sensitivity of F wave and H reflex to changes in motoneuronal excitability. Muscle Nerve 19: 1342–1344
17. Grillner S (1986) Interaction between sensory signals and the central networks controlling locomotion, in lamprey, dogfish and cat. In: Grillner S, Stein PSG, Stuart DG, Forssberg H, Herman RM, (eds) Neurobiology of vertebrate locomotion, vol 45. Wenner-Gren International Symposium Series, pp 505–512
18. Kiehn O (1991) Plateau potentials and active integration in the 'final common pathway' for motor behaviour. Trends Neurosci 14: 68–73
19. Barnes C, Joynt R, Schottelius B (1962) Motoneuron resting potential in spinal shock. Am J Physiol 203: 1113–1116
20. Buller AJ, Eccles JC, Eccles RM (1960) Interactions between motoneurons and muscles in respect of the characteristic speeds of their responses. J Physiol 150: 417–439
21. Burke D (1983) Critical examination of the case for or against fusimotor involvement in disorders of muscle tone. Adv Neurol 39: 133–150
22. Faist M, Mazevet D, Dietz V, Pierrot-Deseilligny E (1994) A quantitative assessment of presynaptic inhibition of Ia afferents in spastics. Differences in hemiplegics and paraplegics. Brain 117: 1449–1455
23. Yang JF, Stein RB (1990) Phase-dependent reflex reversal in human leg muscles during walking. J Neurophysiol 63: 1109–1117
24. Meunier S, Pierrot-Deseilligny E (1998) Cortical control of presynaptic inhibition of Ia afferents in humans. Exp Brain Res 119: 415–426
25. Dengler R, Kossev A, Wohlfahrt K, Schubert M, Elek J, Wolf W (1992) F waves and motor unit size [see comments]. Muscle Nerve 15: 1138–1142
26. Lundberg A (1979) Multisensory control of spinal reflex pathways. Prog Brain Res 50: 11–28
27. Shahani BT, Young RR (1971) Human flexor reflexes. J Neurol Neurosurg Psychiatry 34: 616–627
28. Deschuytere J, DeKeyser C, Deschuttere M, Rosselle N (1983) H reflexes in muscles of the lower and upper limbs in man: identification and clinical significance. Adv Neurol 39: 951–960
29. O'Dwyer NJ, Ada L (1996) Reflex hyperexcitability and muscle contracture in relation to spastic hypertonia. Curr Opin Neurol 9: 451–455
30. Dietz V, Quintern J, Berger W (1981) Electrophysiological studies of gait in spasticity and rigidity. Evidence that altered mechanical properties of muscle contribute to hypertonia. Brain 104: 431–449
31. Edstrom L (1970) Selective changes in the sizes of red and white muscle fibres in upper motor lesions and Parkinsonism. J Neurol Sci 11: 537–550
32. Taylor S, Ashby P, Verrier M (1984) Neurophysiological changes following traumatic spinal lesions in man. J Neurol Neurosurg Psychiatry 47: 1102–1108
33. Aisen ML, Brown W, Rubin M (1992) Electrophysiologic changes in lumbar spinal cord after cervical cord injury [see comments]. Neurology 42: 623–636
34. Dietz V (1997) Neurophysiology of gait disorders: present and future applications. Electroencephalogr Clin Neurophysiol 103: 333–355
35. Ibrahim IK, Berger W, Trippel M, Dietz V (1993) Stretch-induced electromyographic activity and torque in spastic elbow muscles. Differential modulation of reflex activity in passive and active motor tasks. Brain 116: 971–989
36. Dietz V, Wirz M, Jensen L (1997) Locomotion in patients with spinal cord injuries. Phys Ther 77: 508–516
37. Kuhn R (1950) Functional capacitiy of isolated human spinal cord. Brain 73: 1–51
38. Calancie B, Needham-Shropshire B, Jacobs P, Willer K, Zych G, Green BA (1994) Involuntary stepping after chronic spinal cord injury. Evidence for a central rhythm generator for locomotion in man. Brain 117: 1143–1159
39. Bussel B, Roby-Brami A, Azouvi P, Biraben A, Yakovleff A, Held JP (1988) Myoclonus in a patient with spinal cord transection. Possible involvement of the spinal stepping generator. Brain 111: 1235–1245
40. Bussel B, Roby-Brami A, Yakovleff A, Bennis N (1989) Late flexion reflex in paraplegic patients. Evidence for a spinal stepping generator. Brain Res Bull 22: 53–56
41. Dietz V, Colombo G, Jensen L, Baumgartner L (1995) Locomotor capacity of spinal cord in paraplegic patients [see comments]. Ann Neurol 37: 574–582
42. Dietz V, Wirz M, Curt A, Colombo G (1998) Locomotor pattern in paraplegic patients: training effects and recovery of spinal cord function. Spinal Cord 36: 380–390
43. Rossignol S, Barbeau H (1995) New approaches to locomotor rehabilitation in spinal cord injury. Ann Neurol 37: 555–556
44. Dietz V, Colombo G, Jensen L (1994) Locomotor activity in spinal man. Lancet 344: 1260–1263
45. Fung J, Stewart JE, Barbeau H (1990) The combined effects of clonidine and cyproheptadine with interactive training on the modulation of locomotion in spinal cord injured subjects. J Neurol Sci 100: 85–93
46. Wernig A, Muller S, Nanassy A, Cagol E (1995) Laufband therapy based on 'rules of spinal locomotion' is effective in spinal cord injured persons. Eur J Neurosci 7: 823–829
47. Wernig A, Muller S (1992) Laufband locomotion with body weight support improved walking in persons with severe spinal cord injuries. Paraplegia 30: 229–238
48. Grillner S, Deliagina T, Ekeberg O, el Manira A, Hill RH, Lansner A, Orlovsky GN, Wallen P (1995) Neural networks that co-ordinate locomotion and body orientation in lamprey. Trends Neurosci 18: 270–279
49. Dietz V, Nakazawa K, Wirz M, Erni T (1999) Level of spinal cord lesion determines locomotor activity in spinal man. Exp Brain Res 128: 405–409

Correspondence: Prof. Dr. Volker Dietz, ParaCare, Swiss Paraplegic Centre, University Hospital Balgrist, Forchstr. 340, CH – 8008 Zurich, Switzerland. e-mail: dietz@balgrist.unizh.ch

Acta Neurochir (2004) [Suppl] 89: 101–107

Printed in Austria

Lessons from epidemiologic studies in clinical trials of traumatic brain injury

A. Farin and **L. F. Marshall**

Division Neurosurgery, UCSD-Medical Center, San Diego, CA, USA

Summary

Lessions from epidemiological studies

The Clinical Trial Group for Neurosurgery of the University of California San Diego (UCSD) is involved in epidemiological studies and trials of new pharmacological agents in traumatic brain injury. A great number (> 10,000) of patients has been prospectively analyzed forming an integrated database for further purposes. The development of these databases is based on earlier work by the European Neurosurgeons Jennett and Braakmann and the US-Traumatic Coma Data Bank Study. These studies allowed for the development of sophisticated data collection instruments which were used in the international Tirilizad Trials which enrolled over 1,100 patients. A major observation from that trial was that pretreatment hypotension or hypoxia could be unbalanced even in a large two arm blinded study. Another issue of the tirilazad trial was the influence of gender affecting not only outcome but also drug metabolism.

Similar experiences were gathered with the phase-III trial on the competitive NMDA-receptor antagonist selfotel, which interferes with the excitotoxic amino acid glutamate as mediator of secondary brain damage, as ischemia-induced neuronal degeneration. Unfortunately, the trial, already underway, had to be prematurely aborted, since concurrent stroke studies with enrollment of non-intubated patients on low-dose selfotel revealed an increased number of deaths and other adverse events. A retrospective analysis did not confirm that Selfotel was associated with an increased mortality in TBI, but there was also no evidence that the drug was efficacious. A problem here was that a major portion of patients did not have intracranial mass lesions (contusion, subdural haematoma) on CT, questioning whether these had a treatment responsive brain injury.

Both studies on tirilazad or selfotel underscore the significance of well designed and conducted phase-I and -II trials to characterize the pharmacokinetics of the agent, to confirm availability of drug in the brain, and to identify a sufficient number of patients with lesions responding to the drug. A major issue is the blood-brain barrier permeability of the agent under study. Further, the phenomenon of secondary deterioration – *neurological worsening* – turned out as a powerful predictor of poor outcome. The findings and conclusions of both clinical trials (tirilazad, selfotel) were utilized for a subsequent patient study on CP101-606 in consultation with the Pfizer company, the US Brain Injury Consortium, and the San Diego Clinical Trial Group. The patient population was a priori selected towards responsiveness of the brain lesions to the treatment. The major conclusions are

I Development of therapeutic regimens targeted towards the mechanisms of brain injury
II Availability of adequate preclinical data
III Directing treatment towards an appropriate patient population
IV Central gathering and interpretation of the neuroradiological findings
V Monitoring of trial center performance
VI Stratification and pre-trial prognostic analysis for identification of subgroups

Keywords: Traumatic brain injury; clinical drugtrial; tirilazad; selfotel; CP101-606; neurological worsening; brain lesion responsiveness.

Introduction

The Clinical Trials Group in Neurosurgery at the University of California at San Diego (UCSD) has been engaged both in epidemiologic studies and in efficacy trials of new pharmacologic therapies for brain injury over the past 20 years. More than 10,000 patients have been systematically and prospectively studied, permitting the creation of a very large integrated database which not only allows studies of the epidemiology of head injury and potential pharmacological efficacy, but has also enabled us to explore additional views, such as how changes in other types of treatment other than drug therapy have or may influence outcome.

The Traumatic Coma Data Bank (TCDB) served as the first model for very detailed data collection in patients with severe head injury and represented a major effort to utilize computerized data banking techniques to study trends in severe head injury [1]. The Traumatic Coma Data Bank clearly benefitted from the pioneering multinational studies of outcome led by Jennett and Braakman, which primarily focused on the prediction of outcome in patients with severe head injury [2]. The TCDB has reported a number of important observations which are listed in Table 1. The TCDB provided the first detailed analysis of the inter-

Table 1. *Accomplishments and observations of TCDB*

First application of computerized analytical techniques to detailed head injury data
First attempt to temporally relate extracranial events to intracranial events
First clear delineation of relationship of shock to ICP and brain swelling and to outcome
First detailed analysis of traumatic subarachnoid hemorrhage and its influence on outcome [28]
First detailed study of the role of extracranial injuries in determining outcome
First descriptions of patterns of recovery from severe injury
First hint of aberrant regeneration
First demonstration of unacceptable risk in intraventricular monitoring in patients with basilar fractures
Development of a new CT classification of head injury
Trimodal outcome based on age in head injury
Determination of the effects of managing intracranial hypertension in patients with diffuse brain swelling

action of extracranial injuries, hypotension and outcome, and provided a new CT classification of head injury, to name two significant accomplishments [3, 4, 5]. The TCDB also emphasized the influence of traumatic subarachnoid hemorrhage on outcome, following the pioneering work of Wilkins [6, 7], and began to explore the relationship between treatment for varying patterns of brain injury as well as patterns of recovery from severe head injury. Advances in computer technology and the widespread availability of more powerful personal computers allowed subsequent studies to collect even more focused data and to carry out more complex and elegant analyses to characterize a variety of interrelationships the TCDB could not consider.

Analysis of such a comprehensive set of data points permits development of research hypotheses, which can be initially tested in one data subset and subsequently validated or refuted in another. During the past several years, with the assistance of colleagues from around the world, our group has attempted to systematically generate a number of such hypotheses about treatment as well as about methods to improve data collection. We have also sought to identify new criteria of efficacy for clinical trials, including identifying and validating new endpoints for measuring outcome, with the objective of shortening clinical trials. Moreover, in some cases appropriately combining separate data sets may enable certain conclusions to be drawn, which would otherwise remain hidden within a smaller data set. While this may serve as a potentially powerful research strategy, there are substantial limitations which must be understood when combining separately collected data sets.

The tirilazad trial

Tirilazad is an inhibitor of free-radical mediated lipid peroxidation [8]. During Phase I and Phase II trials, it was shown to have a good safety profile and to be effective with experimental models of head injury even in the presence of hypoxia. In 1991, the Clinical Trials Group in Neurosurgery at UCSD began managing an international prospective multicenter trial to study tirilazad's efficacy in moderate and severe head injury. The European/Australian trial included centers with considerable experience in managing severe head injury, in clinical research and in protocol compliance. This trial included 957 patients with severe head injury and 163 with moderate head injury; a significant effect in the full population was not demonstrated, though a significant effect in males with traumatic SAH was noted [9]. Unfortunately, a parallel North American study was terminated before full enrollment was attained because of higher mortality in the treatment group, though this increase was not significant when 6-month outcomes were analyzed [10].

Experience from the TCDB had led trial designers to insist on centralized interpretation of CT scans, which proved extremely valuable in subsequent outcome analysis. Still, the North American tirilazad trial was retrospectively found to be plagued with imbalances in several prognostic entry criteria, including motor scores, pretreatment CT classification and frequency of bilaterally unreactive pupils. Additionally, patients with pretreatment hypotension given placebo had an unexpectedly good outcome, further confounding results [11]. Despite a large sample size and block randomization in the European trial, the frequencies of pretreatment hypotension, hypoxia and epidural hematoma favored outcome in patients treated with placebo [4]. After termination of the Tirilazad trials it was recognized that the agent apparently did not cross the blood-brain barrier in high enough concentrations in the severely head injured [11].

The tirilazad trials also underscored the importance of gender in affecting overall outcome from brain injury and in affecting drug metabolism. The studies of tirilazad in aneurysmal SAH initially demonstrated a substantial difference in outcome based on gender, with males faring substantially better than females [12]. A similar and significant difference in outcome

Table 2. *Lessons from the tirilazad trials*

1.) Avoid collection of non-essential data.
2.) Gender differences may be very important in overall outcome from brain injury and in determining efficacy.
3.) New classification for traumatic subarachnoid hemorrhage (tSAH) and recognition that tSAH is frequent, complex and important in determining outcome.
4.) Strict monitoring of trial centers is essential in pharmacologic trials.
5.) Centralized interpretation of neurological assists in standardizing therapy.
6.) TCDB CT classification of brain damage can reliably predict outcome.
7.) Heterogeneity of head injury populations requires a clear focus in clinical trials.
8.) Muscle relaxants do not influence outcome.
9.) Likelihood of attaining adequate brain tissue levels of drugs in man must be determined before human trials begin.

between men and women in the tirilazad head injury trials was also identified, particularly in women who had also suffered traumatic SAH [2]. In retrospect, unbalanced randomization of traumatic SAH may have acted as an additional confounding factor in the tirilazad trials. It was also retrospectively discovered that women had lower plasma levels of tirilazad, sometimes below the therapeutic range [13], and that metabolism of tirilazad was increased by phenytoin [14]. This is of concern because seizure prophylaxis is common in head injury management in the United States. That women with traumatic SAH had poorer outcomes may have been partly due to the later recognized more rapid metabolism of the drug in females. The fact that tirilazad was shown to have significant efficacy in men with traumatic SAH may indicate that therapeutic concentrations were achieved in appropriate compartments including the microvascular bed and cerebrospinal fluid as a consequence of the traumatic SAH [11]. Table 2 summarizes lessons learned from the tirilazad trials.

Observations from the tirilazad database did enable validation of the traumatic SAH classification developed by Morris in San Diego. Figure 1 describes the classification system and Fig. 2 demonstrates the influence of traumatic SAH on outcome in the tirilazad trials.

Grade:	CT Scan Findings
Grade 0	No evidence of traumatic subarachnoid hemorrhage (tSAH)
Grade 1	tSAH present in only one location
Grade 2	tSAH present in one location with blood filling structure OR tSAH present in two locations without blood filling either structure
Grade 3	tSAH present in two locations, one of which includes tentorium filled with blood
Grade 4	tSAH present in three or more locations, any quantity

Fig. 1. Proposed classification of traumatic subarachnoid hemorrhage

Grade:	Mortality	Favorable Outcome
Grade 0	13%	78%
Grade 1	18%	59%
Grade 2	25%	51%
Grade 3	31%	44%
Grade 4	44%	29%

Fig. 2. Proposed outcome predictability of traumatic subarachnoid hemorrhage

The selfotel trial

The competitive NMDA receptor antagonist selfotel was tested in two multicenter Phase III trials of patients with severe head injury [15] after investigators reported that excessive concentrations of excitatory amino acids, especially glutamate, can lead to secondary damage [16] and further that NMDA antagonists can block ischemia-induced neuronal degeneration [17, 18]. Before full enrollment was attained, however, the trials were stopped due to concern over increased deaths and serious adverse events in two concurrent stroke trials involving unintubated patients receiving much lower doses [19]. Though the head injury data did not show an increased frequency of serious adverse events, the data accumulated by the time the trials were terminated were not promising that efficacy would be demonstrated. Subsequent studies revealed that up to 40 percent of patients enrolled in these trials had no intracranial mass lesions, including focal contusions and acute subdural hematomas, and therefore constituted groups with a low likelihood of excess glutamate release as part of their pathophysiology [20]. Inclusion of such patients without CT evidence of brain damage in this trial and in clinical trials of the severe head injured in general is quite problematic. First, very low mortality in patients without CT evidence of brain damage makes it almost impossible to demonstrate differences in rates of death between placebo and treatment groups. In addition, cognitive and behavioral assessment methods appear to be inadequate to detect favorable or unfavorable influence of therapeutic intervention.

The tirilazad and selfotel examples demonstrate the importance of Phase I and II studies in characterizing pharmocokinetics, demonstrating adequate target organ drug availability, and identifying an appropriate patient population whose pathophysiology matches the drug's mechanism of action. Like tirilazad, selfotel was also found to have poor brain penetration; in head trauma, low cerebral blood flow would impair drug delivery to the brain even more [21]. Without adequate penetration, this competitive NMDA receptor antagonist could not be expected to interfere with the binding of endogenous glutamate to its receptor.

An additional observation from the international selfotel trials was an apparent difference in care among centers in patients with traumatic intraparenchymal hemorrhages. In some institutions these patients underwent early evacuation of such hematomas even if they were of relatively small size, while in others surgery was almost never performed. This difference may well be meaningful in determining outcome because the preliminary analysis suggested that patients with lower GCS scores and larger hematomas fared better when operated on early than patients with smaller lesions and higher GCS scores were the lesion later "blossomed" and required emergent intervention. This is in keeping with our observations based on the same data that neurologic deterioration or neurologic worsening is an extremely powerful predictor of an adverse outcome.

The selfotel trials benefited from being sequenced immediately after the tirilazad trials in that there was better agreement on CT scan interpretation between the central reader and the individual centers than was found in the tirilazad trials. Information collected during the selfotel trials was better focused and more specifically relevant than the broader data set collected during the tirilazad trials. Table 3 summarizes lessons learned from the selfotel trials.

Table 3. *Lessons from the selfotel trials*

1.) Patients without CT evidence of brain damage have outcomes too favorable to detect influences of therapy using present cognitive and behavioral methods.
2.) Adverse events in parallel trials of different diseases (i.e., stroke) should not influence initiation or continuation of head injury trials.
3.) Intercenter differences in care may influence outcome and are difficult to control.
4.) The purported mechanism of action of a drug needs to be taken into account in determining targeted populations.
5.) ICP is a much more powerful determinant of outcome than CPP.
6.) Muscle relaxants do no influence outcome.
7.) Likelihood of attaining adequate brain tissue levels of drugs in man must be determined before human trials begin.

Table 4. *Lessons from the Pfizer trial (ongoing)*

1.) Difficulty in demonstrating therapeutic benefit in Diffuse Injury II population unless SAH or lesion $\geq$ 5 cc present.
2.) Classification of traumatic SAH developed from Tirilazad database validated.
3.) Drug target appropriate and pharmacokinetics confirm appropriate tissue levels in man.

The Pfizer trial

The CP 101-606 trial was designed through consultation between Pfizer, the American Brain Injury Consortium and our group. Much effort was made to limit the cohort of patients to be studied in an attempt to improve the probability of detecting a treatment effect given past experience. In the selfotel trial, it had been observed that patients without CT evidence of significant brain damage had a mortality rate of approximately 5% and a rate of favorable outcome over 75%. Therefore, in the CP 101-606 trial, eligible patients in the Diffuse Injury II CT category had evidence of a lesion at least 5 cc in size and/or SAH. Preliminary analysis of this trial which has now been completed demonstrates a mortality rate of approximately 15% in this specific subgroup, potentially allowing for better detection of a treatment effect.

This trial piloted the use of the extended Glasgow Outcome Scale, or EGOS, in attempt to sharpen the ability to detect differences in outcome which may have been missed by the use of a broader scale such as the GOS. By requiring more structured interview with regard to patient function in a variety of domains it is possible that a more clear differentiation between placebo and treatment groups be detected, if there is a treatment effect. Table 4 summarizes lessons learned from the Pfizer Trial.

Lessons learned from head injury trials

Analysis of outcome data in patients with moderate and severe brain injury has led to several important principles that should be considered when designing future trials so that any possible treatment effect will be demonstrated unequivocally. Future efforts should focus on:

Developing therapeutic regimens targeted toward multiple mechanisms of injury

Multiple mechanisms of brain damage at the cellular level are clearly responsible for the complex nature of head injury. Single treatment allows for the possibility that the therapeutic mechanism being delivered may not adequately address the most critical aspect of patient pathophysiology. Therefore, single treatment is less likely to be efficacious for the total population than either drugs with multiple mechanisms of action or sequential therapy. This reasoning may partly explain why the trials described above failed to show significantly improved outcomes in the total treatment groups. Single agents may be shown to be efficacious only in specific subgroups of head injured patients [22, 23]. Given the complexity of head injury, perhaps efforts should be better focused on characterizing the chronologic sequence of activation of various pathophysiologic mechanisms post injury. These may then serve as appropriate targets for drugs with matched mechanisms of action at various time points post injury.

Performing adequate preclinical studies

Agents must be adequately tested preclinically to determine key information before Phase III trials are initiated. Conclusions about dose-response curves, time window response curves, length of treatment, therapeutic range, target organ drug availability and drug metabolism must be accurately extrapolated from experimental models.

Directing therapy to the appropriate patient population

The head injured population to be studied should have a pattern of brain injury that is amenable to the mechanism of action of the proposed treatment. It is inappropriate for example, to use a drug that is an NMDA receptor antagonist with little or no change in glutamate concentrations in the population being studied.

Centralized interpretation of neuroradiologic imaging studies

Centralized readings of the CT scans is essential to ensure the inclusion and exclusion of patients within the trial. It also serves as a marker of the quality of treatment provided in each center for two reasons. First, in general poor CT interpretation at a site tends to be associated with failure to comply with the protocol. The pattern of brain injury seen on CT clearly influences treatment. Thus, it is essential that center performance be stringently controlled in such trials.

Monitoring of trial centers' performance by experienced monitors

Good monitoring can limit the inherent variability in such trials even when protocols are strictly defined and enforced.

Employing stratification and prognostic equations and making available to authorities pre-analyses identification of sub-groups

Despite strict inclusion and exclusion criteria, the head injured patients included in clinical trials remain heterogeneous, especially with respect to their mechanisms of damage, pathophysiology and clinical condition. Even with randomization and enrollment > 800, imbalances in the distribution of prognostic variables, including age, Glasgow Coma Scale scores, pupillary reactivity, CT classification and pretreatment hypotension or hypoxia, are still quite possible. Given the heterogeneity of head injured patients, clinical trials should classify baseline risk variables from the outset and stratify patients accordingly so that frequencies of baseline risk variables are similar between the treatment and placebo groups. Some argue that patients should also be randomized by the probability that they will achieve a certain recovery [24, 25, 26, 27]. Prediction of outcome soon after injury would identify patients whose clinical condition plays a strong role in determining outcome as opposed to patients whose outcome is less certain – this latter "intermediate risk" group would enable investigators to obtain results more reflective of the therapeutic effect rather than a dominant prognostic effect. Prognostic equations would also more accurately characterize risk distribution between treatment groups and therefore help ensure better comparability of groups rather than simply comparing frequencies of prognostic variables across groups. During the data analysis phase, multivariable analysis, including regression analysis, can adjust for imbalanced baseline characteristics and yield findings that apply to patients with a specific risk profile.

Conclusion

The creation of computer databases containing essential information about head injured patients and computer analysis of these large data sets has greatly facilitated hypothesis generation, enabled development of new methods to systematically classify the heterogeneous head injury population, and permitted recognition of how several key factors affect outcome. The experience we have gained conducting clinical trials has enabled our colleagues and us to draw a number of significant conclusions about how to modify trial design so that efficacy can be properly assessed. In order to derive meaningful conclusions from a heterogeneous population, several points must be considered. Adequate preclinical studies must be performed before human trials begin. Therapy must be directed to an appropriate patient population. Neurological imaging studies should be centrally interpreted. Trial centers must be monitored to ensure protocol adherence. Stratification and prognostic equations, as well as early identification of subgroups, will result in more robust findings. It has become additionally apparent that although the primary impact in head injury remains the most significant determinant of outcome, several secondary biochemical factors interact to produce varying patterns of recovery. It is unlikely that a pharmacologic treatment aimed simply at one neurochemical derangement that occurs in brain injury will be sufficient to improve the outcome of the millions of people worldwide who suffer brain injury each year. More promising are single therapies which have multiple mechanisms of action or sequential therapies ordered based on our present understanding of the pathophysiology of this major public health problem.

References

1. Foulkes MA, Eisenberg HM, Jane JA, Marmarou A, Marshall LF, and The Traumatic Coma Data Bank Resarch Group (1991) The Traumatic Coma Data Bank: design, methods, and baseline characteristics. Report on the Traumatic Coma Data Bank. J Neurosurg (S) 75: 8–13
2. Jennett B, Teasdale G, Galbraith S, Pickard J, Grant H, Braakman R, Avezaat C, Maas A, Minderhoud J, Vecht CJ, Heiden J, Small R, Caton W, Kurze T (1977) Severe head injury in three countries. J Neurol Neurosurg Psychiatry 40: 292–298
3. Marshall LF, Gautille T, Klauber MR, Eisenberg HM, Jane JA, Luerssen TG, Marmarou A, Foulkes MA (1991) The outcome of severe closed head injury. Report on the Traumatic Coma Data Bank. J Neurosurg (S) 75: 28–36
4. Vollmer DG, Torner JC, Jane JA, Sadovnic B, Charlebois D, Eisenberg HM, Foulkes MA, Marmarou A, Marshall LF (1991) Age and outcome following traumatic coma: why do older patients fare worse? Report on the Traumatic Coma Data Bank. J Neurosurg (S) 75: 37–49
5. Marshall LF, Marshall SB, Klauber MR, Clark MVB, Eisenberg HM, Jane JA, Luerssen TG, Marmarou A, Foulkes MA (1991) A new classification of head injury based on computerized tomography. Report on the Traumatic Coma Data Bank. J Neurosurg (S) 75: 14–20
6. Wilkins RH, Alexander JA, Odom GL (1968) Intracranial arterial spasm: a clinical analysis. J Neurosurg 29: 121–134
7. Wilkins RH, Odom GL (1970) Intracranial arterial spasm associated with craniocerebral trauma. J Neurosurg 32: 626–633
8. Hall ED, Yonkers PA, McCall JM, Braughler JM (1988) Effects of the 21-aminosteroid U-74006F on experimental head injury in mice. J Neurosurg 68: 456–461
9. Marshall LF, Maas AIR, Marshall SB, Bricolo A, Fearnside M, Iannotti F, Klauber MR, Lagarrigue J, Lobato R, Persson L, Pickard JD, Piek J, Servadei F, Wellis GN, Morris GF, Means ED, Musch B (1998) A multicenter trial on the efficacy of using tirilazad mesylate in case of head injury. J Neurosurg 89: 519–525
10. Straw RN, Means ED, Kitt TM, Murray FT, Ogrinc FG, Leonard LB, Ruppel PL (1995) Preliminary efficacy and safety results from Protocol P/2700/0017. Tirilazad mesylate in the treatment of acute head injury (North American study) – technical report. Pharmacia & Upjohn Co., Kalamazoo, MI
11. Maas AIR, Steyerberg EW, Murray GD, Bullock RB, Baethmann A, Marshall LF, Teasdale GM (1999) Why have recent trials of neuroprotective agents in head injury failed to show convincing efficacy? A pragmatic analysis and theoretical considerations. Neurosurgery 6: 1286–1298
12. Kassell NF, Haley EC, Apperson-Hansen C *et al* (1996) A randomized double-blind, vehicle-controlled trial of tirilazad mesylate in patients with aneurismal subarachnoid hemorrhage: a cooperative study in Europe/Australia/New Zealand. J Neurosurg 84: 221–228
13. Fleishaker JC, Hulst-Pearson LK, Peters GR (1995) Effect of gender and menopausal status on the pharmacokinetics of tirilazed mesylate in healthy subjects. Am J Ther 2: 553–560
14. Fleishaker JC, Straw RN, Cross CJ (1997) Pharmacokinetics of tirilazad and U-89678, an active reduced metabolite, following acute head trauma in adults. J Pharm Sci 86: 434–437
15. Morris GF, Bullock R, Marshall SB, Marmarou A, Maas A, Marshall LF (1999) Failure of the competitive N-methyl-D-aspartate antagonist Selfotel (CGS 19755) in the treatment of severe head injury: results of two phase III clinical trials. The Selfotel Investigators. J Neurosurg 91(5): 737–743
16. Hayes RL, Jenkins LW, Lyeth BG (1992) Neurotransmitter mediated mechanisms of traumatic brain injury: Acetylcholine and excitatory amino acids. J Neurotrauma [Suppl] 1: 173–187
17. Chen MH, Bullock R, Graham DI, Miller JD, McCulloch J (1991) Ischemic neuronal damage after acute subdural hema-

toma in the rat: Effects of pretreatment with a glutamate antagonist. J Neurosurg 74: 944–950
18. McIntosh TK, Vink R, Soarez H, Hayes R, Simon R (1989) Effects of the N-methyl-D-aspartate receptor blocker MK-801 on neurologic function after experimental brain injury. J Neurotrauma 6: 247–259
19. Davis SM, Albers GW, Diener HC, Lees KR, Norris J (ASSIST Steering Committee) (1997) Termination of acute stroke studies involving selfotel treatment. Lancet 349: 332
20. Bullock R, Zauner A, Woodward JJ, Myseros J, Choi SC, Kaura SC, Ward JD, Marmarou A, Young HF (1998) Factors affecting excitatory amino acid release following severe human head injury. J Neurosurg 89: 507–518
21. Hogan MJ, Takizawa S, Hakim AM (1995) In vitro binding of nimodipine and CGs 19755 to rat brain in focal cerebral ischemia. Exp Neurol 134: 56–63
22. European Study Group on Nimodipine in Severe Head Injury (1994) A multicenter trial of the efficacy of nimodipine on outcome after severe head injury. J Neurosurg 80: 797–804
23. Grumme T, Baethmann A, Kolodziejczyk D, Krimmer J, Fischer M, von Eisenhart Rothe B, Pelka R, Bennefeld H, Pollauer E, Kostron H, Leheta F, Necek S, Neeser G, Sachsenheimer W, Sommerauer J, Verhoeven F (1995) Treatment of patients with severe head injury by triamcinolone: a prospective, controlled multicenter clinical trial of 396 cases. Res Exp Med (Berl) 195: 217–229
24. Braakman R, Gelpke GJ, Habbema JDF, Maas AIR, Minderhoud JM (1980) Systematic selection of prognostic features in patients with severe head injury. Neurosurgery 6: 362–370
25. Choi SC, Barnes TY (1996) Predicting outcome in the head injured patient. In: Narayan RK, Wilberger JE, Povlishock JT (eds). Neurotrauma. McGraw-Hill, New York, pp 779–792
26. Jennett B, Teasdale GM, Braakman R, Minderhoud J, Knill-Jones R (1976) Predicting outcome in individual patients after severe head injury. Lancet 1: 1031–1034
27. Narayan RK, Greenberg RP, Miller JD, Enas GG, Choi SC, Kishore PR, Selhorst JB, Lutz HA III, Becker DP (1981) Improved confidence of outcome prediction in severe head injury. J Neurosurg 54: 751–762
28. Eisenberg HM, Gary HE Jr, Aldrich EF, Saydjari C, Turner B, Foulkes MA, Jane JA, Marmarou A, Marshall LF, Young HF (1990) Initial CT findings in 753 patients with severe head injury: a report from the NIH Traumatic Coma Data Bank. J Neurosurg 73(5): 688–698

Correspondence: Prof. Dr. L. F. Marshall, M.D., Ph.D., Chief, Division Neurosurgery, 200 West Arbor Drive, San Diego, CA 92103, USA.

Acta Neurochir (2004) [Suppl] 89: 109–112

Printed in Austria

The MRC CRASH trial – a large, simple randomised trial of steroids in head injury

J. Wasserberg on behalf of the CRASH trial collaborative group

Department of Neurosurgery, Queen Elizabeth Hospital, Birmingham, United Kingdom

Summary

CRASH (Corticosteroid randomisation after significant head injury) is a prospective multi-centre randomised double blind study of methylprednisolone versus placebo in mild, moderate and severe head injury. Patients are eligible up to 8 hours from injury. To date the CRASH trial has recruited 9000 patients. The trial is recruiting from 200 hospitals in 50 countries with another 100 centres planning to join the trial. The target for recruitment is 20,000 patients by 2006. The trial is wholly funded by the Medical Research Council of Great Britain and is multidisciplinary, involving doctors and nurses from a range of specialities. A recent systematic review of corticosteroids in head injury demonstrated a risk of death in the corticosteroid treated group 2% lower than in the control group. The 95% confidence interval ranges from a 6% lower mortality to a 2% higher mortality. This result is compatible with there being no real benefit, but it is also compatible with there being a small benefit of a few percent. An improvement in mortality of 2% would theoretically save 10,000 lives per 500,000 patients treated. The global impact of such a treatment effect would be significant as the number of head injuries world-wide continues to rise.

Keywords: Randomised controlled trial; head injury; corticosteroid.

Introduction

Head injury is the main contributor to trauma related mortality. Overall mortality in trauma patients is about three times higher in patients with head injury compared to those without, with a reported mortality of 14–30 per 100,000 of the population per year. In developed countries approximately 100–300 per 100,000 of the population are at risk of suffering a head injury per year with a slightly higher incidence in less developed countries. By the year 2020 it is estimated that motor vehicle accident related trauma will be the third highest global disease burden and the second in the developing world [9]. Other common causes of head injury worldwide are falls, alcohol intake and gunshot wounds.

Head injuries can be classified by conscious level using the Glasgow coma scale (GCS) which has a lowest score of 3 corresponding to a deep coma to a highest of 15 which corresponds to a normal conscious level. Using the score obtained when the patient is first admitted to hospital, head injuries can be classified into mild (GCS 13–15), moderate [9–12] and severe [3–8] head injury.

The outcome for all three types of head injury has been improved over the last 40 years due to improvements in pre-hospital care and trauma systems, the universal availability of computerised tomographic scanning (CT) and improvements in intensive care. Most of the interventions used in head injury do not have a strong evidence base and indeed a recent evidence based review of such interventions did not find class A evidence for benefit from any of the treatments used [4]. The use of corticosteroids in head injury remains quite common despite an absence of evidence for it's efficacy. Steroids are used in 64% of US trauma centres [6], 49% of UK intensive care units [9] and in 14% of neurosurgical intensive care units in the United Kingdom [5].

So far all the randomised trials of corticosteroids have been small: the largest included only a few hundred patients and even in aggregate they have involved only about 2000 patients. Combining all previous trials the risk of death in the corticosteroid treated group is approximately 2% lower than in the control group (Aggregate mortality 37% in corticosteroid group v 39% in control group, odds ratio 0.91, 95% confidence interval 0.72–1.11). The 95% confidence interval runs from 6% lower to a 2% higher mortality [1]. The overall result is compatible with there being no real benefit but it is easily compatible with there being a small benefit of a few percent. However the existing trials are too small to demonstrate or refute either possibility. Even a modest reduction in mortality would represent a significant increase in lives saved. For instance a 2% reduction in mortality and a similar reduction in disability would theoretically save 10,000 lives and prevent 10,000 disabilities per 500,000 patients treated. At the present time the use of steroids varies widely between clinicians, hospitals and countries.

Experimental basis for the trial

Laboratory studies of animal models of head injury and clinical studies in human spinal cord injury support a possible benefit of corticosteroids in head injury.

High dose methylprednisolone has been shown to reduce post-traumatic neuronal degeneration and improve outcome in animal head injury models. Hall demonstrated that 30 mg/kg of methylprednisolone enhanced neurological recovery in mice that were subjected to moderately severe brain injury when given five minutes post injury [8]. To date, there have been only two small randomised trials of high dose (30 mg/kg) methylprednisolone in head injury [7, 11]. In both there was a non-significant reduction in the risk of death in the methylprednisolone treated group. However, because the trials were small, the effectiveness of high dose methylprednisolone in the treatment of head injury remains uncertain (pooled risk difference 3% lower mortality, 95% confidence interval 14% lower to 9% higher).

Results from animal studies also suggest that early administration of corticosteroid is important for maximal effect. Because axonal disruption after acute central nervous system trauma does not occur for several hours, there may be an early phase when neurological deficit is reversible [12]. Administration of corticosteroids within 8 hours has also been shown to be important in acute spinal cord injury [2, 3]. However, the administration of corticosteroids in many of the existing trials in head injury may have been outside this window of opportunity.

Corticosteroids in human spinal cord injury

Evidence of benefit from corticosteroids in acute human spinal cord injury has renewed interest in their role in brain injury. The Second US National Acute Spinal Cord Injury Study (NASCIS 2) compared 24 hours of methylprednisolone or naloxone with placebo in 333 patients with acute spinal cord injury [2]. At six months, patients receiving methylprednisolone within eight hours of injury had greater improvement in motor function and sensation to pinprick and fine touch than in patients treated with placebo [2]. A subsequent trial (NASCIS 3) of methylprednisolone in acute spinal cord injury demonstrated slightly more neurological recovery in patients receiving corticosteroids for 48 rather than 24 hours of treatment [3]. On the basis of these results high dose methylprednisolone is now widely used in the management of acute spinal cord injury.

The CRASH trial

The CRASH trial (Corticosteroid randomisation after significant head injury) is a large simple randomised trial of steroids in head injury [12]. The trial aims to recruit 20,000 patients to receive either methyprednisolone or placebo intravenously within 8 hours of injury. Any patient older than 16 years with any reduction of conscious level as measured by the Glasgow coma score is eligible for randomisation (Fig 1. Protocol box). Outcome is measured using the Glasgow Outcome score at 14 days and six months using a simple questionnaire. The trial is fully supported by the publicly funded British Medical Research Council and receives no funding from the pharmaceutical industry. A pharmaceutical company, Pfizer is supplying the trial drugs, methylprednisolone or placebo free of charge. The start up phase of the trial begun in April 1999 and the trial was officially launched in December 2000. 1203 patients have been recruited from 66 centres in 20 countries with 250 centres planning to join the trial. It is now the largest randomised controlled trial of steroids in head injury and recruitment data show a satisfactory increase in recruitment rates and addition of new collaborating centres world-wide.

Issues of consent

The eligibility for randomisation in the CRASH trial includes any reduction in conscious level. By definition therefore the patient is not able to make an informed decision about whether to enter the trial. Issues regarding consent depend on the laws of individual countries and must be approved by both national and local ethics committees. In England patients are ran-

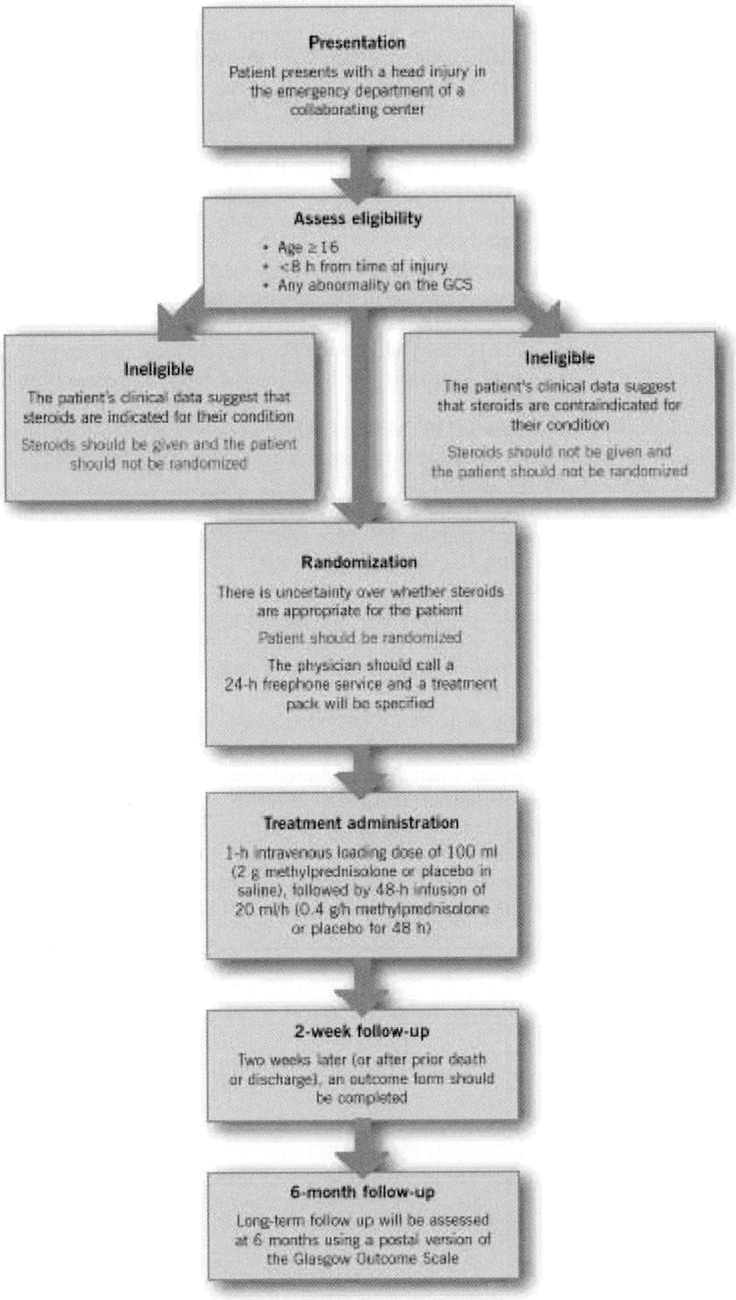

Fig. 1. Inclusion of patients in the CRASH trial

domised and treated as soon as possible after admission. Relatives are informed as soon as possible and given an information leaflet and an opportunity to ask questions. They are asked if they have any objections to the trial continuing for the full 48 hours of steroid administration. In other countries informed consent from a relative has to be obtained prior to randomisation. Each collaborating centre must seek local guidance and approval for the method of consent used.

More centres are required that routinely admit head injured patients and hospitals in any country are encouraged to apply. The trail will run until 2005 and is powered to detect a potential positive benefit from steroids of 2%.

Conclusion

Review of the literature therefore demonstrates an *absence of evidence* for any benefit from corticosteroids in head injury but does not confirm a widely held anecdotal view that there is *evidence of no benefit [1]*. This is an important distinction and underlies the ethical basis for this trial. A negative result from the trial would support the discontinuation of a potentially harmful treatment whereas a positive result would support the use of a beneficial treatment. Further information on the CRASH trial can be found on the internet at www.crash.lshtm.ac.uk.

References

1. Alderson P, Roberts I (1997) Corticosteroids in acute traumatic brain injury: systematic review of randomised controlled trials. BMJ 314: 1855–1859
2. Bracken MB, Shepard MJ, Collins WF, Holford TR, Young W, Baskins DS, Eisenberg HM, Flamm E, Leo-Summers L, Maroon J (1990) A randomised, controlled trial of methylprednisolone or naloxone in the treatment of acute spinal cord injury. Results of the Second National Acute Spinal Cord Injury Study. New Engl J Med 322(20): 1405–1411
3. Bracken MB, Shepard MJ, Holford TR, Leo-Summers L, Aldrich EF, Fazl M, Fehlings MG, Herr DL, Hitchon PW, Marshall LF, Nockels RP, Pascale V, Perot PL Jr, Piepmeier J, Sonntag VK, Wagner F, Wilberger JE, Winn HR, Young W (1998) Methylprednisolone or tirilizad mesylate admnistration after acute spinal cord injury: 1-year follow up. Results of the third national acute spinal cord injury randomised controled trial. J Neurosurg 89(5): 699–706
4. Bullock R, Chesnut RM, Clifton G, Ghajar J, Marion DW, Narayan RK, Newell DW, Pitts LH, Rosner MJ, Wilberger JW (1996) Guidelines for the Management of severe head injury. Brain Trauma Foundation. Eur J Emerg Med 3(2): 109–127
5. Crimmins DW, Palmer JD (2000) Snapshot view of emergency neurosurgical head injury care in Great Britain and Ireland. J Neurol Neurosurgery Psychiatry 68: 8–13
6. Ghajar J, Hariri RJ, Narayan RK, Iacono LA, Firlik K, Patterson RH (1995) Survey of critical care management of comatose head injured patients in the United States. Crit Care Med 23(3): 560–567
7. Giannotta SL, Weiss MH, Apuzzo MLJ, Martin E (1984) High dose glucocorticoids in the management of severe head injury. Neurosurgery 15: 497–501
8. Hall ED (1985) High dose glucocorticoid treatment improves neurological recovery in head injured mice. J Neurosurg 62: 882–887
9. Jeevaratnam DR, Menon DK (1996) Survey of intensive care of severely head injured patients in the United Kingdom. BMJ 312: 944–947
10. Murray CJL, Lopez AD (1997) Alternative projections of mortality and disability by cause 1990–2020: Global Burden of Disease Study. Lancet 349: 1498–1504
11. Stubbs DF, Stiger TR, Harris WR (1989) Multinational controlled trial of high-dose Methylprednisolone in moderately severe head injury. In: Capildeo R (ed) Steroids in diseases of the central nervous system. John Wiley & Sons, Chichester, pp 163–168
12. Yates D, Roberts I (2000) Corticosteroids in head injury. It's time for a large simple randomised trial. CRASH trial management group. Corticosteroid randomisation after significant head injury. (Editorial) BMJ 321(7254): 128–129

Correspondence: Jonathan Wasserberg, Department of Neurosurgery, Queen Elizabeth Hospital, Edgbaston, Birmingham B15 2TH, United Kingdom. e-mail: crash@lshtm.ac.uk.

Acta Neurochir (2004) [Suppl] 89: 113–118

Printed in Austria

Clinical trials in traumatic brain injury: current problems and future solutions

A. I. R. Maas[1], **A. Marmarou**[4], **G. D. Murray**[2] and **E. W. Steyerberg**[3]

[1] Department of Neurosurgery, Erasmus University Medical Center Rotterdam, Rotterdam, The Netherlands
[2] Public Health Sciences, University of Edinburgh, Edinburgh, Scotland, UK
[3] Department of Public Health, Erasmus University Medical Center Rotterdam, Rotterdam, The Netherlands
[4] Department of Neurosurgery, Virginia Commonwealth University, Richmond, USA

Summary

Over the past decade many neuroprotective agents have been developed with the hope of being able to improve outcome in patients with traumatic brain injury. Unfortunately, none of the phase III trials performed have convincingly demonstrated efficacy in the overall population. A common misconception is that consequently these agents are ineffective. Such has not been proven and some trials show evidence of efficacy in subgroups of the population studied. The negative results, as reported in the overall population, may in part be caused by specific aspects of the TBI population, as well as by aspects of clinical trial design and analysis. Clinical trials in TBI pose several complicated design issues. Methodological challenges relate particularly to heterogeneity of the population and to outcome assessment. Heterogeneity pertains both to the range of pathologies included in TBI, and to prognostic factors, each causing specific problems. Mechanistic and/or prognostic targeting, as well as possibilities for covariate adjustment, are suggested as possible solutions to deal with the problems of heterogeneity.

The aim in most trials was to demonstrate a 10% absolute improvement in favorable outcome in patients with head injury. This may be considered overoptimistic and unrealistic in relation to the heterogeneous patient population. Specific problems are further incurred by the use of the dichotomized Glasgow Outcome Scale as primary outcome measure. Optimal statistical power may expected to be present when the point of dichotomization results in a 50:50 distribution of outcome categories. It is proposed to differentiate the point of dichotomization according to prognostic risk profile, in order to maintain statistical power.

Solutions described may be expected to enhance chances of demonstrating benefit of potentially effective neuroprotective agents in future studies. The complexity of problems occurring in clinical trial design and analysis in TBI is such that a strong and sustained multidisciplinary input and effort is required from all experts involved in the field of neurotrauma.

Keywords: Traumatic brain injury; clinical trials; outcome; prognosis; neuroprotection.

Overview

Traumatic brain injury (TBI) is a heterogeneous disease, encompassing a wide range of pathologies. The main components are axonal injury, ischemia, focal contusions with perifocal edema, intracranial hematomas and brain swelling, either due to edema or vascular engorgement. The primary injury initiates subsequent secondary events, which may conceptually be divided into two components: secondary damage and secondary insults. Secondary damage follows activation of selfpropagating destructive biochemical and immunological processes. Systemic insults (e.g. hypotension, hypoxia) and intracranial insults (e.g. mass lesions, raised intracranial pressure) potentiate secondary damage. The central concept that underlies evaluation of neuroprotective therapy in TBI is prevention and treatment of secondary damage [14]. The past decade has been characterized by great advances in our understanding of pathophysiologic processes, causing secondary brain damage [19, 24]. The increased understanding of the importance of such mechanisms has prompted the development of neuroprotective agents aimed at ameliorating such mechanisms. Neuroprotective agents may be classified into three categories:

- agents inhibiting pathophysiologic processes, which in excess may lead to secondary brain damage;
- agents stimulating protective pathways;
- agents and therapies aimed at promoting regeneration.

Phase III randomized clinical trials in the field of TBI have primarily concentrated on agents and therapies inhibiting pathophysiologic processes. Table 1 provides an overview of the major phase III trials, conducted in the past 10 to 15 years. We note that most

Table 1. *Overview of large phase III trials, conducted in head injury*

Study	Mechanism targeted	Agent	Study population	Start of treatment	Year of study	Status	Published	Result
Triamcinolone Steroid trial	various intracerebral processes	Triamcinolone	severe head injury, not further defined	≤4 hours	1985–1990	completed	1995 (9)	no significant effect
HIT I	Calcium mediated damage	Nimodipine	not obeying commands	24 hours	1987–1989	completed	1991 (2)	no significant effect
HIT II	Calcium mediated damage	Nimodipine	not obeying commands	12 hours of not obeying commands within 24 hours of injury	1989–1991	completed	1994 (7)	no significant effect overall population
HIT III	Calcium mediated damage	Nimodipine	tSAH	≤12 hours	1994	completed	1996 (11)	significant reduction in unfavorable outcome
PEGSOD	Free radical damage	PEGSOD	GCS ≤ 8	within 8 hours	1993–1995	completed	1996 (26)	no significant difference
Tirilazad domestic trial	Lipid peroxidation	Tirilazad	GCS ≤ 8: 70–80% GCS 9–12: 20–30%	≤4 hours	1991–1994	terminated	no	no significant effect reported
Tirilazad international trial	Lipid peroxidation	Tirilazad	GCS ≤ 8: 85% GCS 9–12: 15%	≤4 hours	1992–1994	completed	1998 (18)	no significant effect
Eliprodil study	Glutamate excitotoxicity	Eliprodil	GCS 4–8	≤12 hours	1993–1995	completed	no	no significant effect reported
Selfotel	Glutamate excitotoxicity	Selfotel	GCS 4–8	≤8 hours and within 4 hours of admission	1994–1996	terminated	1999 (20)	no significant effect
Cerestat	Glutamate excitotoxicity	Aptiganel	GCS 4–8 GCS 3 if pupils reactive	≤8 hours	1996–1997	terminated	no	no significant effect
Sandoz/Novartis	Glutamate excitotoxicity	D-CPP-ene	not obeying commands, 1 reactive pupil	≤12 hours	1995–1997	completed	in preparation	no significant effect reported
CBF targeted management	Cerebral ischemia	–	Motor score ≤ 5	≤12 h	1995–1998	completed	1999 (21)	No significant effects on outcome Decreased incidence of desaturation episodes Increased incidence of ARDS
NABIS Hypothermia	Various intracerebral processes	–	GCS 3–8 Motor score 1–5	≤6 h	1994–1998	halted	2001 (5)	no effects on outcome reduced incidence of ICP > 30
Bradycor	Bradykinin (β2 receptor) antagonist	CP-0127	GCS 3–8	≤8 h	1996	terminated	1999 (17)	12% improvement in fav. outcome (p = 0,26)
Parke Davis	Calcium channel blocker	SNX-111	GCS 4–8	≤12 h	1997–1998	terminated	–	higher mortality
Pfizer	Glutamate excitotoxicity	CP-101606	GCS 4–8	≤8 h	1997–2000	completed Sept. 2000	–	awaited
HIT IV	Calcium mediated damage	Nimodipine	GCS < 15 + traumatic subarachnoid hemorrhage	≤12 h	1997–1999	completed	in preparation	no significant effect

trials showed no statistically significant effect of the treatment that was investigated.

Mechanisms causing secondary brain damage are complex and interrelated. Uncertainty exists as to when and which pathological mechanisms are active in a specific patient and whether such mechanisms may initially be protective, but when present in excess, turn detrimental. It may therefore be presumed a very difficult task to demonstrate efficacy of a therapy, targeted at one isolated pathophysiologic pathway in the overall population of TBI. Indeed, none of the phase III trails have convincingly demonstrated efficacy in the overall study population (Table 1) [13]. The primary endpoint in these trials was the Glasgow Outcome Scale, dichotomized as unfavorable or favorable. In most trials the hypothesis was that a therapy or neuroprotective agent investigated would increase the absolute proportion of patients with favorable outcome by at least 10%. Such an effect may not have been proven at this predetermined level, but conversely neither has inefficacy been proven. An increase in favorable outcome has been observed in many trials, albeit that these increases have not been statistically significant. For example, the HIT I trial on Nimodipine showed an 8% relative improvement [2] and the HIT II trial a 4% abolute improvement in favorable outcome in treated patients [7]. In the PEGSOD trial a 6% absolute improvement in the trichotomized GOS was noted [26]. In the Triamcinolone trial a 5% absolute increase in good recovery was observed in patients on active treatment [9]. The Bradycor trial showed a 12% absolute improvement in favorable outcome at six months ($p = 0.26$) [17].

In other trials a beneficial effect was noted in subgroups, or in a more targeted population [7, 9, 11, 18]. In a combined analysis, we estimated an overall odds ratio of 0.90 as the pooled effect of neuroprotective agents, using a random effect meta-analysis method to incorporate between study heterogeneity [13]. This effect is similar to the results of the meta-analysis on the results of all identified corticosteroid trials in head injury, both published and unpublished, concluding that a 2% absolute reduction in mortality is plausible [1].

It would appear that at least some trials show an indication of efficacy, either in the overall population or in subgroups. The lack of statistical significance in the overall population may be due to a combination of overly optimistic expectations and insensitive methodology. The sad result is that further development of many of these drugs has been halted and that uncertainty remains concerning a more modest treatment benefit which could still be of great clinical relevance.

Factors, which may have influenced the "negative" results of phase III trials in TBI

Various factors have been proposed which may have contributed to the failure of head injury trials to demonstrate convincing efficacy in the overall population. These factors include uncertainty about validity and robustness of preclinical data and data from phase II trials, problems in translating results from the experimental studies to clinical practice, uncertainty whether the pathophysiologic mechanisms that are targeted are indeed active in individual patients, and if so at what time after injury, uncertainty about the therapeutic window and inadequacies in clinical trial design and analysis [4, 13, 14, 25]. Clinical trials conducted in TBI pose several complicated design issues. Methodological challenges relate particularly to the heterogeneity of the population and to outcome assessment.

Heterogeneity in the TBI population

The influence of heterogeneity is dependent on sample size. A crucial factor in many older trials has been inadequate sample size. It has been argued that problems due to heterogeneity may be obviated in large mega-trials [6]. However, in view of the complexity of trials in the field of TBI, uncertainty concerning risks involved in the use of new non-approved agents, and the cost involved, such mega-trials may not be considered feasible. Moreover, mega-trials still suffer from some of the problems of heterogeneity, i.e. that an analysis of the unadjusted treatment effect may be considered biased [8] and inefficient [22]. Mechanistic and prognostic targeting, as well as covariate adjustment may be a satisfactory alternative to deal with the effects of heterogeneity. In mechanistic targeting the study should preferably be aimed at those patients in whom the pathophysiologic mechanism, targeted by the agent under investigation is active, or alternatively towards a population with a specific type of pathology, in which the mechanisms targeted preferentially occur (e.g. focal lesions). Effects of mechanistic targeting can be examined hypothetically in simulation studies, such as reported by Machado *et al.* [16] as uncertainty exists as to which pathophysiologic mechanisms occur in individual patients. It was shown that mechanistic targeting, benefiting patients with focal injuries, might permit reduction in sample size by half, assuming that the pathophysiologic mechanism targeted is active in all patients.

In prognostic targeting the trial is targeted to a population in which no strong prognostic effect is present, and consequently realistic chances exist for demonstrating potential efficacy, e.g. to patients with an intermediate prognosis. Prognostic targeting has seldom been applied to studies in the field of TBI. Braakman *et al.* [3] reporting on a megadose steroid trial showed that although on analysis of the six month outcome no difference was found between groups, in patients with an intermediate prognosis (e.g. probability of survival between 0.3 and 0.9) an 8% reduction in mortality was noted in the steroid-treated patients. A prediction tree model was employed in the SNX-111 trial to stratify patients on enrolment differentiating between a good and poor stratum.

The effect of prognostic targeting on statistical power has been studied in unselected series of TBI [16], but not as yet in trial populations. In this study it was demonstrated that targeting therapy to patients with an intermediate prognosis was shown to allow a potential reduction of sample size by 30%. Benefits of mechanistic or prognostic targeting were more pronounced in modeling studies, including both severe and moderate patients and less pronounced thought still substantial when based on patients with severe injuries. These studies were performed on the EBIC core data study, which is an unselected series. It is conceivable that the stricter selection of patients enrolled in clinical trials may reduce the advantages of prognostic targeting.

The application of covariate adjustment in the context of randomized clinical trials is a topic of debate among biostatisticians and trialists. One might simply argue that randomization guarantees balance with respect to observed and unobserved covariates. Although this is on average true, imbalances in covariates may well occur in relatively small studies. Moreover, small imbalances in important covariates may lead to substantial and undesired differences between treatment groups. Other advantages include that the effect of treatment is estimated on a more individualized level [12] and that an increase in statistical power can be achieved [22]. Some methodological studies recommend the application of a predefined set of covariates for adjustment of treatment effect. Such procedures have been followed in trials in the cardiovascular area, for instance the GUSTO-III trial (n = 15,000), which had an adjusted analysis specified as the primary statistical analysis in the trial protocol [10]. This approach is however uncommon in the analysis of clinical trials in general, as well as in TBI. The application of adjusted analysis in TBI trials merits further study, since considerable advantages may be achieved with respect to correction of imbalance, more individualized interpretation of a treatment effect, and higher statistical power [23].

Outcome assessment

The primary endpoint in phase III trials in TBI has been the Glasgow Outcome Scale (GOS) evaluated after six months. A characteristic of the GOS is that it is an ordinal scale, but this possible advantage has not been fully exploited. To our knowledge an ordinal analysis has only been specified in the Eliprodil study, but the results of this trial have not been reported. The GOS has been criticized for being insensitive, especially in patients with more favorable outcomes. This insensitivity may be one of the reasons for inability to detect a significant benefit in TBI trials. Insensitivity is further caused by the accepted practice of dichotomizing the GOS to produce two groups: favorable outcome (moderate disability, good recovery) and unfavorable outcome (dead, vegetative, severe disability). Optimal statistical power would be expected to be present when the point of dichotomization results in a 50:50 distribution of outcome categories. The expected distribution will change according to varying enrollment criteria between studies, and patients with different risk profiles may be identified within the population under investigation. Potentially the point of dichotomization could be differentiated according to the prognostic risk profile in order to maintain optimal statistical power. When considering differentiation of dichotomy according to risk profile, "survival" may be an appropriate endpoint for patients at high risk of poor outcome. In contrast, "good recovery" may be an appropriate endpoint for patients at low risk. The applicability of such a "sliding dichotomy", as first proposed for analysis in stroke studies, was examined by us using the data from the Tirilazad trials. The analysis was performed in all patients included in the Tirilazad trials with complete data available to allow calculation of the prognostic score, and with six month GOS recorded. Table 2 shows the outcome distribution in relation to quartiles of baseline risk. This analysis indicates that the point of optimal di-

Table 2. *Optimal dichotomization in relation to prognostic banding; arrows indicate optimal point of dichotomy*

	N	Unfav (%)	GR	MD	SD	V	D
Best prognosis	362	14%	↓ 63%	23%	8.5%	0.3%	5.6%
Better prognosis	362	34%	46%	↓ 20%	14%	3.3%	17%
Worse prognosis	362	59%	26%	14%	↓ 20%	5.0%	35%
Worst prognosis	362	78%	10%	11%	17%	9.7%	↓ 52%
Total	1448	46%					

chotomization (e.g. 50:50 distribution) shifts substantially across prognostic groups. Preliminary analysis indicates a possible gain of 30% in statistical power in the use of such an approach.

Alternatively, an ordinal analysis, exploiting the full GOS, may be considered. However, in a modeling study we could only demonstrate a theoretical benefit of such an approach. No increase in power was however observed in the analysis of previously performed trials [13].

Conclusions

Mechanistic and/or prognostic targeting, as well as covariate adjustment should be considered for dealing with effects of heterogeneity in TBI patients. Also the primary endpoint might be differentiated according to initial prognostic risk profile. The complexity of problems occurring in clinical trial design and analysis is such that a strong and sustained input and effort is required from all experts involved in the field of neurotrauma.

Acknowledgements

Grant support was provided by NIH NS 42691.

References

1. Alderson P, Roberts I (1997) Corticosteroids in acute traumatic brain injury: systematic review of randomised controlled trials. Br Med J 314: 1855–1859
2. Bailey I, Bell A, Gray J, Gullan R, Heiskanan O, Marks PV, Marsh H, Mendelow DA, Murray G, Ohman J *et al* (1991) A trial of the effect of nimodipine on outcome after head injury. Acta Neurochir (Wien) 110: 97–105
3. Braakman R, Schouten HJ, Blaauw-van Dishoeck M, Minderhoud JM (1983) Megadose steroids in severe head injury. Results of a prospective double-blind clinical trial. J Neurosurg 58: 326–330
4. Bullock R, Lyeth BG, Muizelaar JP (1999) Current status of neuroprotection trials for traumatic brain injury: lessons from animal models and clinical studies. Neurosurg 45: 207–220
5. Clifton GL, Miller ER, Choi RN, Levin HS, McCauley S, Smith KR *et al* (2001) Failure of effect of induction of hypothermia after acute brain injury. N Engl J Med 344: 556–563
6. Dickinson K, Bunn F, Wentz R, Edwards P, Roberts I (2000) Size and quality of randomised controlled trials in head injury: review of published studies. Brit Med J 320: 1308–1311
7. The European Study Group on Nimodipine in severe head injury (1994) A multicenter trial of the efficacy of nimodipine on outcome after severe head injury. J Neurosurg 80: 797–804
8. Gail MH, Wieand S, Piantadosi S (1984) Biased estimates of treatment effect in randomised experiments with non linear regressions and omitted covariates. Biometrika 71: 431–444
9. Grumme T, Baethmann A, Kolodziejczyk D, Krimmer J, Fischer M, von Eisenhart Rothe B, Pelka R, Bennefeld H, Pollauer E, Kostron H *et al* (1995) Treatment of patients with severe head injury by triamcinolone: a prospective, controlled multicenter clinical trial of 396 cases. Res Exp Med 195: 217–229
10. The Global Use of Strategies to Open Occluded Coronary Arteries (GUSTO III) Investigators (1997) A comparison of reteplase with alteplase for acute myocardial infarction. N Engl J Med 337: 1118–1123
11. Harders A, Kakarieka A, Braakman R (1996) Traumatic subarachnoid hemorrhage and its treatment with nimodipine. German tSAH Study Group. J Neurosurg 85: 82–89
12. Hauck WW, Anderson S, Marcus SM (1998) Should we adjust for covariates in nonlinear regression analyses of randomized trials? Control Clin Trials 19: 249–256
13. Maas AIR, Steyerberg EW, Murray GD, Bullock R, Baethmann A, Marshall LF, Teasdale GM (1999) Why have recent trials of neuroprotective agents in head injury failed to show convincing efficacy? A pragmatic analysis and theoretical considerations. Neurosurg 44: 1286–1298
14. Maas AIR, Dearden M, Servadei F, Stocchetti N, Unterberg A (2000) Current recommendations for neurotrauma. Current Opinion in Crit Care 6: 281–292
15. Maas AIR (2000) Assessment of agents for the treatment of head injury. Problems and pitfalls in trial design. CNS Drugs 13(2): 139–154
16. Machado SG, Murray GD, Teasdale GM (1999) Evaluation of designs for clinical trials of neuroprotective agents in head injury. European Brain Injury Consortium. J Neurotrauma 16: 1131–1138
17. Marmarou A, Nichols J, Burgess J *et al* (1999) Effects of the bradykinin antagonist bradycor^{tm} (deltibant, cp-0127) in severe

traumatic brain injury: results of a multi-center, randomized, placebo-controlled trial. J Neurotrauma 16: 431–444
18. Marshall LF, Maas AIR, Marshall SB, Bricolo A, Fearnside M, Iannotti F, Klauber MR, Lagarrigue J, Lobato R, Persson L, Pickard JD, Piek J, Servadei F, Wellis GN, Morris GF, Means ED, Musch B (1998) A multicenter trial on the efficacy of using tirilazad mesylate in cases of head injury. J Neurosurg 89: 519–525
19. Marshall LF (2000) Head injury: recent past, present, and future. Neurosurg 47: 546–561
20. Morris GF, Marshall SB, Bullock R *et al* and the Selfotel Investigators (1999) Failure of the competitive NMDA antagonist Selfotel (CGS 19755) to improve outcome after severe head injury. J Neurosurg 91: 737–743
21. Robertson CS, Valadka AB, Hannay HJ, Contant CF, Gopinath SP, Cormio M *et al* (1999) Prevention of secondary ischemic insults after severe head injury. Crit Care Med 27: 2086–2095
22. Robinson LD, Jewell NP (1991) Some surprising results about covariate adjustment in logistic regression models. Int Statist Rev 58: 227–240
23. Steyerberg EW, Bossuyt PM, Lee KL (2000) Clinical trials in acute myocardial infarction: should we adjust for baseline characteristics? Am Heart J 139: 745–751
24. Teasdale GM, Graham DI (1998) Craniocerebral trauma: protection and retrieval of the neuronal population after injury. Neurosurg 43: 723–737
25. Teasdale GM, Maas A, Iannotti F, Ohman J, Unterberg A (1999) Challenges in translating the efficacy of neuroprotective agents in experimental models into knowledge of clinical benefits in head injured patients. Acta Neurochir (Wien) [Suppl] 73: 111–116
26. Young B, Runge JW, Waxman KS, Harrington T, Wilberger J, Muizelaar JP, Boddy A, Kupiec JW (1996) Effects of pegorgotein on neurologic outcome of patients with severe head injury. A multicenter, randomized controlled trial JAMA 276: 538–543

Correspondence: Dr. A. I. R. Maas, Erasmus University Medical Center Rotterdam, Department of Neurosurgery, Dr. Molewaterplein 40, 3015 GD Rotterdam, The Netherlands. e-mail: airmaas@erasmusmc.nl

Acta Neurochir (2004) [Suppl] 89: 119–123

Printed in Austria

Prospective documentation and analysis of the pre- and early clinical management in severe head injury in Southern Bavaria at a population based level*

A. Wirth, A. Baethmann, A. Schlesinger-Raab and Study Group of BMBF-Research Consortium Neurotraumatology and Neuropsychological Rehabilitation: J. Assal, S. Aydemir, M. Bayeff-Filloff, J. Beck, A. Belg, A. Boscher, D. Chapuis, H.-G. Dietz, J. Döffinger, W. Eisenmenger, W. Gerstner, W.-E. Göbel, P. Große, T. Grumme, L. Gutermuth, D. Hölzel, F. Höpner, R. Huf, H. Jaksche, U. Jensen, M. Kettemann, R. Ketterl, U. Kirmayer, D. Kolodziejcyk, W. Köstler, J. Kuznik, C. Lackner, G. Lenz, H. Lochbihler, C. Lumenta, S. Martin, A. Preisz, G. Prokscha, G. Regel, H. Reischl, H.-J. Reulen, F. Rothmeier, D. Sackerer, S. Schneck, L. Schweiberer, F. Sommer, H.-J. Steiger, E. Stolpe, W. Stummer, P. Tanner, A. Trappe, J. v. Twickel, P. Ueblacker, W. Wambach, P. Wengert, and **S. Zimmerer**

Summary

Treatment of patients suffering from severe head injury is so far restricted to general procedures, whereas specific pharmacological agents of neuroprotection including hypothermia have not been found to improve the outcome in clinical trials. Albeit effective, symptomatic measures of the preclinical rescue of patients (i.e. stabilization or reestablishment of the circulatory and respiratory system) or of the early clinical care (e.g. prompt diagnosis and treatment of an intracranial space occupying mass, maintenance of a competent circulatory and respiratory system, and others) by and large constitute the current treatment based on considerable organizational and logistical efforts. These and other components of the head injury treatment are certainly worthwhile of a systematic analysis as to their efficacy or remaining deficiencies, respectively. Deficits could be associated with delays of providing preclinical rescue procedures (e.g. until intubation of the patient or administration of fluid). Delays could also be associated in the hospital with the diagnostic establishment of intracranial lesions requiring prompt neurosurgical intervention.

By support of the *Federal Ministry of Education and Research* and under the auspices of the *Forschungsverbund Neurotraumatology*, University of Munich, a prospective system analysis was carried out on major aspects of the pre- and early clinical management at a population based level in patients with traumatic brain injury. Documentation of pertinent data was made from August 1998 to July 1999 covering a catchment area of Southern Bavaria (5.6 mio inhabitants). Altogether 528 cases identified to suffer from severe head injury (GCS ≤ 8 or deteriorating to that level within 48 hrs) were enrolled following admission to the hospital and establishment of the diagnosis. Further, patients dying on the scene or during transport to the hospital were also documented, particularly as to the frequency of severe head injury as underlying cause of mortality. The analysis included also cases with additional peripheral trauma (*polytrauma*). The efficacy of the logistics and organization of the management was studied by documentation of prognosis-relevant time intervals, as for example until arrival of the rescue squad at the scene of an accident, until intubation and administration of fluid, or upon hospital admission until establishment of the CT-diagnosis and commencement of surgery or transfer to the intensive care unit, respectively.

The severity of cases studied in the present analysis is evident from a mortality of far above 40% of cases admitted to the hospital, which was increased by about 20% when including prehospital mortality. The outcome data notwithstanding, the emerging results demonstrate a high efficacy of the pre- and early clinical management, as indicated by a prompt arrival of the rescue squad at the scene, a competent prehospital and early clinical management and care, indicative of a low rate of avoidable complications. It is tentatively concluded on the basis of these findings that the patient prognosis is increasingly determined by the manifestations of *primary brain damage* vs. the development of *secondary complications*.

The article is based on a publication in European Surgical Research, 34, 2002.

Introduction

Severe head trauma including damage of the brain still is the most frequent cause of morbidity and mortality up to approximately 45 years. The most important sequelae of general trauma is severe head injury, which is determining the outcome of trauma victims, so far particularly affecting the male population of younger age. The financial burden are enormous of severe head injury aside from the personal tragedy and suffering. Losses involve not only the futile expenses for education and professional training but also that the future income of the victim is lost in addition to the

* Supported by BMBF-Research Consortium *Neurotraumatology und Neuropsychological Rehabilitation Munich.*

medical expenses including those for the lifelong care in patients with severe disability.

In Germany, approximately 280,000 patients are annually admitted to hospitals with the diagnosis of *brain injury*, fortunately enough mostly of mild or moderate nature only. This notwithstanding ca. 5% of cases can be considered as severe according to the worldwide accepted definition of a neurological deficit of ≤8 points of the *Glasgow Coma Score* for 6 to 24 hours after trauma, or deterioration to that level within 48 hours. Based on the *Federal Bureau of Statistics*, Wiesbaden, Germany, 7,705 patients were dying in 1999 from severe head injury in the Federal Republic of Germany (*ICD 10 diagnosis*: (a) *intracranial injuries,* (b) *skull fracture*), which may translate into a frequency of *severe traumatic brain injury per year* of 12,630 [1]. From this figure, an incidence of 1,200 patients with severe disabilities per annum can be extrapolated, which yearly is increasing the prevalence of severely disabled already surviving as dependants in specific care facilities or at home.

The treatment of patients with traumatic brain injury encompasses a comprehensive package of measures, not only consisting of the preclinical resuscitation and management, but also of the early clinical diagnostic procedures and treatment with all its logistical and organizational support. Their effective administration requires great competence and skills, among others of the emergency physicians and preclinical rescue personnel at the scene, but also of the services providing clinical care. Further, a high level of organization and logistics of the preclinical rescue is necessary together with a dense availability of trauma centers with neurosurgical competence including intensive care facilities. Last but not least, head injury patients require sophisticated neuropsychological rehabilitation – a formidable challenge.

Specific pharmacological agents affording neuroprotection to prevent the development of *secondary brain damage* have not been found so far to be effective in prospective clinical trials, notwithstanding that a variety of methods have a remarkable therapeutical potential under experimental conditions. The problem of why these agents and procedures, e.g. interfering with neuroexcitotoxic glutamate effects, formation of O_2-derived free radicals, and other mechanisms causing *secondary brain damage* (i.e. an additional loss of brain parenchyma) has been extensively analysed [2]. It is hoped that conclusions and suggestions emerging from this and former metaanalyses eventually lead to solutions out of the present deadlock, providing novel design and concepts for future trials to more convincingly elucidate, whether experimentally efficient methods of neuroprotection are useful for the treatment of severe head injury patients. Until then, the currently available treatment and management armamentarium should continuously be subjected to a critical analysis as to its efficacy and remaining deficits.

This, actually is the purpose of an elaborate *System Analysis* of the BMBF-Research Consortium *Neurotraumatology and Neuropsychological Rehabilitation* supported by the Federal Ministry of Education and Research in Germany [3]. Details of this analysis include documentation of the course of events, so to say from the time point of an accident together with the patients' state, e.g. level of consciousness, visible injuries, complications, as arterial hypotension or hypoxia from aspiration, etc. In addition, rescue measures at the scene, as intubation, infusions, and others were protocolled. The present investigations were carried out on a population based level, representing a catchment area in Southern Bavaria of ca. 5.6 Mio inhabitants to collect epidemiologically valid data also with regard to the incidence of severe head injury and its outcome.

In the course of these investigations it became obvious that outcome findings published in the past quite often are influenced by the purpose of a given study, consequently the in- and exclusion criteria adjusted to the specific objectives of a given trial. With such a procedure a major number of patients may be eliminated and ignored, often those who are dying within 24 hrs after the traumatic insult. Another point of the present investigation was to assess the frequency of severe head injury cases, dying *prior to hospital admission* for which practically no information is made available by former investigations. Reliable data are missing also on the frequency of the severely disabled survivors, which often constitute a group of young male victims remaining dependent for the rest of their life in rehabilitation facilities or at home. Quantitative information on the annual incidence of this outcome, however, is important for the planning of necessary institutional capacities and, thereby, of interest for insurance organizations.

With regard to the assessment of the present management quality, a major point was to gather information on the time-course of care with onset at the scene of an accident until arrival of the emergency squad, intubation and stabilization of the patient, as e.g. recognizable from normalisation of the blood pressure, and others. Further, the time point of hospital admission was of interest, the subsequent establishment of the CT-diagnosis, and – last but not least – conclusion of acute care, as defined by the beginning of a neurosurgical operation or transfer to the intensive care unit. An important objective was also concerned with the remaining significance of *secondary brain damage* for the outcome of patients with severe head injury.

As known, the prognosis in traumatic brain injury is largely determined by two factors (a) *nature and severity of the primary lesion* of the brain produced at the moment of an insult and (b) the subsequent *sequelae resulting in secondary damage of the brain – the additional loss of brain parenchyma.* The distinction is not of academic interest but clinically highly significant, as only the complications leading to secondary brain damage might be influenced by the management and treatment. This explains, why a better understanding of underlying mechanisms is so important, since a further reduction of the morbidity and mortality in severe head injury can only be expected from their more efficient prevention and treatment. This not only demonstrates the great significance of progress in the patient management and care at all levels, beginning at the scene of an accident to more effectively inhibit the development of *avoidable complications*, but also of the availability of neuroprotective measures and agents proving effective in clinical trials.

In this context, it is quite clear that a severely head injured patient is at high risk, not only during the preclinical rescue period with usually less than optimal conditions of resuscitation and stabilization, but also during the early clinical phase as indicated by the fact that the mortality peak occurs at the first/second day after trauma. Whereas it is easily understood that a multitude of complications, as aspiration, internal bleeding causing cardiovascular failure and other instabilities are liable to put the patient at risk during the *prehospital rescue period*, problems remain after the patient has been admitted to the hospital. Studies of *avoidable complications* in children succumbing from head injury in England have shown that dangerous events are taking place during the clinical care period approximately 2–3 times more frequently than during the preclinical rescue [4]. A prospective risk assessment was made under the coordination of the late J. D. Miller, Univ. Edinburgh/Scotland in severe head injured patients. Important physiological parameters, as *intracranial pressure, blood pressure, blood gases* and others were densely monitored during an intrahospital transfer of patients, from the intensive care unit to CT scanning, among others. Accordingly, in no less than 83% of these manoeuvres the patients' homeostasis was severely impaired as concluded, for example from an increase of the *intracranial pressure* and *arterial blood pressure*, or a decrease of the *systemic blood pressure* together with *arterial hypoxia* [5]. This demonstrates that even under well controlled stable conditions in a maximal care hospital, complications – being avoidable or not – evolve which may support the development of *secondary brain damage*.

Study objectives

In view of the above considerations an in-depth analysis of the major components of the management and treatment of patients with head injury, beginning at the scene as soon as possible after a traumatic insult, and including the early clinical care phase appeared to be mandatory. For that purpose, a *Study Group* was established and coordinated by the University of Munich with support by the BMBF-Research Consortium *Neurotraumatology and Neuropsychological Rehabilitation.* Its mission was to systematically document and collect pertinent data to assess the efficacy of the present care system (i.e. management, logistics, organization, etc.). The analysis was carried out in collaboration with more than 30 hospitals in Munich and the other larger cities in the catchment area and organizations, as the *Red Cross*, emergency services including the dispatch centers for rescue vehicles and helicopters, *fire brigades*, and – last but not least – the *Department of Forensic Medicine*, the *Institute for Surgical Research*, and *Institute for Biometrics and Epidemiology* of the University of Munich.

For the population based investigations patients were recruited, if they were matching the following inclusion criteria: neurological deficit of ≤8 points of the *Glasgow Coma Scale* at the site of an accident or deterioration to that level within 48 hrs. With regard to the geographical definition of the catchment area, patients suffering an insult *within* this area, but receiving treatment *outside* or, *vice versa* were excluded, as well as those without pathology in the CT scan, and finally children younger than two years. The *Study Apparatus* was organized as a network of the ten dispatch centers in the catchment area, including four helicopter stations in: Munich, Ingolstadt, Kempten, Traunstein, and forensic medical institutions in Munich, Kempten, Memmingen, Ingolstadt and Augsburg.

Most important, *documentation assistants* (young physicians at the beginning of their medical training) were hired and strategically distributed within the catchment area, i.e. in Munich, Augsburg, Ingolstadt, Murnau, Traunstein, Vogtareuth and Altötting. Each colleague was establishing a close communication network with approximately 5 to 10 regional hospitals by daily telephone interviews and frequent site visits from where newly admitted patients with head injury were reported. Thereby, a close follow-up of the patients' course was afforded during the acute documentation period of the first 12 days after the accident.

The documentation network was coordinated by the *Study Center* localized at the *Institute for Surgical Research* of the Klinikum of the University of Munich-Großhadern. All relevant data and information was collected in a data bank. The *Study Center* was coordinated by biostatisticians, who not only were devising the software for the data bank and subsequent statistical analysis, but also carrying out a daily back-up of the data flow, utilizing advanced biometrical procedures including for the assessment of risk factors for the outcome.

Of all patients finally recruited for clinical documentation, the majority were seen at the site of an accident and transported by a ground based ambulance provided with an emergency physician. One third of all patients admitted to hospitals received emergency treatment at the scene by a helicopter rescue staff also including an emergency physician. The most frequent mechanism of injury were jumps and falls of victims >55 years old, followed by traffic accidents involving cars, pedestrians, bicycle- and motorcycle riders. In the group of cases dying at the scene prior to hospitalization, suicidal railway accidents and gun shot wounds were representing the most frequent causes of injury, followed by traffic accidents, jumps and falls.

Arrival of the rescue squad with a physician at the scene was accomplished in the majority of cases within the legally required period after alarm. Rescue and resuscitation for stabilization of the patient was carried out according to the "*stay and play*" philosophy. All the potentially outcome-relevant time periods, e.g. until intubation of patients, admission to the hospital, establishment of the CT-diagnosis, or conclusion of acute care were documented in order to evaluate and assess the time-course of the preclinical- and early clinical management. *Conclusion of acute care* was identified as the time-point, when the patient was delivered to the intensive care unit or to the operation theatre for surgery. As reference, the time of the first alarm of the dispatch center in a given case from the scene of an accident was taken, since the time of an accident proper almost always is unavailable. In the current study, about 20% of patients were secondarily admitted to the final care hospital providing neurosurgery from a primary general trauma hospital. This was extending the period of acute care by approximately 100%, a potentially important delay which was analysed as to its impact on the final outcome.

During the preclinical rescue phase important complications were documented, as respiratory distress, apnea, tracheal aspiration, tachy- or bradycardia, occurrence, severity, and duration of arterial hypotension (systolic blood pressure < 80 mmHg). The latter is a major risk factor of poor outcome in severe head injury [6]. In addition, all pertinent measures of the preclinical management were protocolled, such as infusion of fluid, intubation, and ventilation with additional oxygen, analgo-sedation, and others. In this context, tracheal clearing, cardiac massage, defibrillation, or thoracic draining may be mentioned in addition. In patients with additional polytrauma with a higher risk of arterial hypotension, the effectivity of normalising arterial blood pressure was documented by repeated measurements of the systemic blood pressure at the scene immediately upon arrival of the emergency squad and continued until admission to the hospital.

The outcome of the hospitalised patients was studied at 3, 6, or 12 months after the accident. The prognosis of severe head injury was assessed with and without the cases dying prior to hospital admission. Analysis of the outcome by inclusion of the prehospital mortality is reflecting more appropriately the overall fatality from severe head injury as compared to many clinical analyses reported in the literature. Quite often, these are limited to the outcome of hospitalised patients sometimes even under exclusion of those dying within 24 hrs after trauma for a stratification of the patient population in drug trials. With inclusion of the prehospital fatalities, the overall mortality was increased by nearly 30% of the intrahospital mortality, with a correspondingly low fraction of cases with good outcome categories.

In conclusion, documentation of the course of patients with severe head injury was carried out for analysis of the management, care, and organization, beginning at the scene of an accident and continuing with a dense protocol during the first 12 days at the hospital. Outcome of the patients was assessed by using the *Glasgow-Outcome-Scale* [7] at 3, 6, and 12 months. Such an analysis has to the best of our knowledge not been performed so far on a prospective basis with documentation of the patients course utilizing a dense network for data gathering. By this approach it is expected that novel information is provided on the persisting role of *secondary brain damage* for the outcome in severe head injury, and the remaining significance of *avoidable complications*. Since patients dying prior to hospitalisation were subjected to autopsy at a high frequency, the contribution of severe head injury to the prehospital mortality for the first time could also be reliably analysed. The findings from the current analysis, particularly the assessment of prevailing risk factors provide a solid basis for considerations concerning potentially necessary improvements of the organization and management. A management at its best possible level, however, is a major requirement for the successful conduct of clinical trials on novel neuroprotective agents, as the patient outcome must not be influenced by avoidable complications leading to secondary brain damage.

Acknowledgment

The secretarial assistance for preparation of this manuscript by Helga Kleylein and Pia Handke is gratefully acknowledged.

References

1. Sterbefälle 1999 nach ausgewählten Todesursachen, Altersgruppen und Geschlecht, Statistisches Bundesamt Wiesbaden. 1999; Fachserie 12, Reihe 4
2. Maas AIR, Steyerberg EW, Murray GD, Bullock R, Baethmann A, Marshall LF, Teasdale GM (1999) Why have recent trials of neuroprotective agents in head injury failed to show convincing efficacy? A pragmatic analysis and theoretical considerations. Neurosurgery 44: 1286–1298
3. Lehr D, Baethmann A and Study Group: Reulen H-J, Steiger H-J, Lackner Ch, Stummer W, Wirth A, Hölzel D, Stolpe E, Assal J, Belg A, Schrödel M, Müller N, Ueblacker P, Chlistalla A, Schneider G, Schweiberer L, Dietz H-G, Trappe A, Göbel W-E, Jaksche H, Messner V, Grumme Th, Wenger P, Müller H, Döffinger J, Lumenta Ch, Gerstner W, Proschka G, Sackerer D, Höfner F, Eisenstein T, Lenz G, Preisz A, Rothmeier F, Kirmayer U, Böhme M, Horak W, Weess Th (1997) Management of patients with severe head injury in the preclinical phase: a prospective analysis. J Trauma: Injury, Infection, Critical Care 42: S71–S75
4. Sharples PM, Storey A, Aynsley-Green A, Eyre JA (1990) Avoidable factors contributing to death of children with head injury. Brit Med J 300: 87–91
5. Andrews PJD, Piper IR, Dearden NM, Miller JD (1990) Secondary insults during intrahospital transport of head injured patients. Lancet 335: 327–330
6. Marmarou A, Anderson RL, Ward JD, Choi SC, Young HF, Eisenberg HM, Foulkes MA, Marshall LF, Jane JA (1991) Impact of ICP-instability and hypotension and outcome in patients with severe head trauma. J Neurosurg 75: S59–S66
7. Jennett B, Bond M (1975) Assessment of outcome after severe brain damage: a practical scale. Lancet 1: 480–484
8. Wirth A, Baethmann A, Schlesinger-Raab A and Study Group of BMBF-Research Consortium Neurotraumatology and Neuropsychological Rehabilitation: Assal J, Aydemir S, Bayeff-Filloff M, Beck J, Belg A, Boscher A, Chapuis D, Dietz H-G, Döffinger J, Eisenmenger W, Gerstner W, Göbel W-E, Große P, Grumme Th, Gutermuth L, Hölzel D, Höpner F, Huf R, Jaksche H, Jensen U, Kettemann M, Ketterl R, Kirmayer U, Kolodziejcyk D, Köstler W, Kuznik J, Lackner Ch, Lenz G, Lochbihler H, Lumenta Ch, Martin S, Preisz A, Prokscha G, Regel G, Reischl H, Reulen H-J, Rothmeier F, Sackerer D, Schneck S, Schweiberer L, Sommer F, Steiger H-J, Stolpe E, Stummer W, Tanner P, Trappe A, v. Twickel J, Ueblacker P, Wambach W, Wengert P, Zimmerer S (2002) Prospective system analysis of the pre- and early hospital care in severe head injury in Bavaria at a population based level. In: Baethmann A, Enders G, Krombach F, Plesnila N (eds) Surgical research – a discipline at the interface of the basic sciences and the clinic. Europ Surg Res 34(1–2): 42–46

Correspondence: A. Baethmann, Institute for Surgical Research, Klinikum of University of Munich, 81366 Munich, Germany. e-mail: baethman@icf.med.uni-muenchen.de

Author Index

Index of Keywords